Climbing Fit

CLIMBING FIT

Martyn Hurn & Pat Ingle

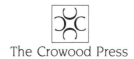

The Crowood Press

First published in 1988 by
The Crowood Press
Ramsbury, Marlborough,
Wiltshire SN8 2HE

Reprinted 1988, 1989

British Library Cataloguing in Publication Data

Hurn, Martyn
  Climbing fit.
  1. Physical fitness   2. Mountaineers – Health and hygiene
  I. Title   II. Ingle, Pat
  613.7'1   RC1220.M6
  ISBN 1 85223 111 4

Typeset by Chippendale Type, Otley, West Yorkshire.
Printed in Great Britain by Redwood Burn Ltd, Trowbridge

Dedicated to Jimmy Jewell

Acknowledgements

Many people have helped us with this book but the following climbers deserve special mention for their patience with the photography and their openness about their training methods: Stevie Haston, Ron Fawcett, Freda Lowe, Anita Jones, Steve Long, Jimmy Jewell, Johnny Dawes, Nicky Wright, Anna Wood, Ray Wood, Matthew Ingle, Janet Palmer, Gerry Moffat, Nick Warner, Caroline Tickle, and Harry Lock. We must also thank Malcolm Griffiths for his photographs and Dr Lew Hardy and Dr John Fazey for their expert opinions.

Contents

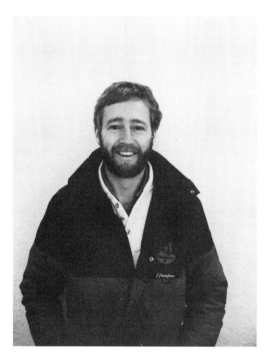

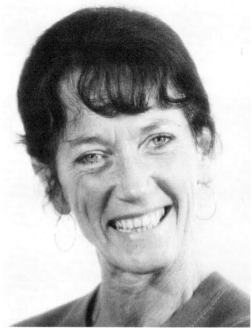

Martyn Hurn has travelled the world, to the Himalayas, North and South America and Africa, in search of new climbing experiences. He has worked as a qualified mountaineering instructor for 10 years, most recently at the National Centre for Mountain Activities in North Wales. He is also a member of the British Association of Ski Instructors, and a coach for the English Ski Council.

Pat Ingle is a specialist fitness trainer with 28 years of climbing experience. A qualified PE teacher, she has lectured in gymnastics at the University College of North Wales, and is the fitness coach for the Welsh ski team. One of her current projects is to instigate training clinics for the climbers of North Wales.

Introduction

Climbing, whether it be rock-gymnastics or Alpinism allows a variety of styles and techniques to succeed. It is this very variety that adds to the uniqueness of the sport and yet allows men and women of all shapes and sizes to succeed at their chosen levels. Training is not new to our sport but never before has it had the following it has today. However, the varied nature of climbing and climbers makes it very difficult to design the perfect fitness programme. For this reason, the following pages will explain some of the theory behind the various elements and offer a number of different programmes you can follow. This should help you to adapt a programme to your own situation.

This, we feel, is the crux of training for climbing. In order to design a proper programme an individual must understand how his body functions, what the requirements are of his particular style and therefore which areas of training need greater emphasis. For example, if you are able to cope with short bursts of very strenuous climbing but tire quickly on the more sustained routes then you should concentrate on working on your endurance. As you proceed through the initial chapters and gain a greater understanding of how your body works, you should be able to narrow down your individual requirements even more closely.

Recently, in the desire for excellence, many top climbers have suffered training injuries, the reasons for which are not always clear. We feel sure that a greater understanding amongst climbers of the mechanisms of training has to be the first step towards reducing the incidence of these injuries. As you will have gathered from the above, the idea of a perfect programme for all climbers will in our opinion always be unattainable because of the variables involved, but do not be daunted by our approach and the need to understand more. In fact by understanding what is actually happening to their bodies many athletes gain a greater degree of motivation. This knowledge will also allow you to listen to your body more clearly and this is vital if you are to get the most out of your training and reduce the chances of injury.

Training, of course, is not for everybody, indeed some climbers will find that the regime of a properly structured training programme interferes with the very freedom that climbing offers them. We make no attempts to persuade you one way or the other, we merely wish to help those of you who do train or who wish to train, to do so in the most constructive and safest of ways. Furthermore, training is not the preserve of those at the top end of the sport – anybody, no matter what standard they are climbing at, can benefit from a well-designed programme, and we hope that you will all find something of value to you in the following pages.

1 The Body

Your body is a complex organism. It is capable of tremendous work-loads and of very skilful actions but it can easily be damaged by inappropriate training. The purpose of this chapter is to explain in relatively simple terms how certain parts of the machine work and what can go wrong with it. By educating yourself in this way you should be able to prevent many injuries and train more effectively so that all the hard work you put into your training is used to the best advantage.

BONES AND JOINTS

The human skeleton performs five major functions and is made up of about 206 bones, which vary considerably in both shape and size. Bones start developing before birth and continue until children are in their late teens. Research suggests that exercise in young children can be beneficial, but over-use can be detrimental – young climbers must therefore be particularly careful about training and should only do so under the guidance of a fully-trained sports coach. A good athletics coach will, even without any knowledge of our sport, be able to help the young climber to develop a programme that will not cause them severe problems later in life.

Functions of the Bones and Joints

1. Supporting the body's soft tissues and organs.
2. The bones together with the joints and muscles provide lever systems that enable movement to take place.
3. They provide protection for a number of organs.

4. The red bone marrow within the bone manufactures blood cells.
5. If insufficient calcium is being absorbed from our food then the body can draw on the reserves within the bones.

The bones are linked together by the joint systems of the body; the majority of these are freely movable and are known as *synovial joints*. Good joint mobility is essential to good climbing and an understanding of the structure of joints may help you prevent unnecessary injuries to them, which in turn might reduce their mobility.

The joint's surface is designed to allow a particular range of movement and is covered with a layer of cartilage which is hard wearing, smooth and thus friction-free. The joint is held together by a capsule which is vital to maintaining the joint's stability. The inside of this capsule is lined by the *synovial membrane* which secretes a lubricating fluid into the joint. There is normally only a small amount of this fluid present, but if the membrane is inflamed then more fluid is released and the joint becomes swollen and sore. The *ligaments*, white fibrous tissues that run between the ends of the joints, also help to hold the joint stable. If they are torn, this may lead to permanent instability of the joint.

Some joints have cartilaginous structures within them, which perform a number of different functions such as reducing friction and absorbing shock. They also improve the congruency of the joints, especially when their size increases during a 'warm-up.' Other lubricating devices are the *bursae*. These are small flat sacs lined with a synovial membrane which, as in the joint, secretes fluid into the sac. The sacs are situated at points where friction might occur such as between muscles and tendons. They

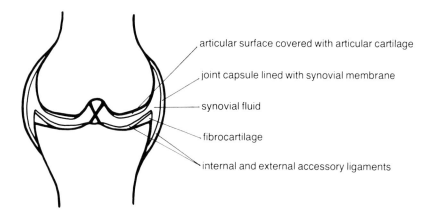

articular surface covered with articular cartilage

joint capsule lined with synovial membrane

synovial fluid

fibrocartilage

internal and external accessory ligaments

Fig 1 A typical joint.

can become inflamed, which will cause painful swelling. In order to accommodate the changing size of the joint capsule that will occur with movement, small fat pads are distributed around the margins of the joint: these too can become inflamed and painful.

The mobility of a joint is reliant on a number of factors, such as the condition of its internal structure, and the natural restrictions that occur with any particular joint. The muscles also have a limiting effect – normally there is a good interplay between opposing muscle groups, but if a movement is made too quickly into the extreme range of movement, the muscle will automatically retract in an effort to protect the joint. Research suggests that there can be an increase of up to 20 per cent in mobility if the ambient temperature is in the region of 110°F (43°C), and an equally dramatic decrease in temperatures below 65°F (18°C). Not only do high temperatures help mobility but they also reduce the chance of injury. Unless we exercise regularly and include mobility as part of our overall routine then we will lose mobility with age. Women tend to be, probably for anatomical reasons, more flexible than men.

Joints can also suffer from fatigue. Experiments have shown that the stretch receptors in ligaments do, under stress, complain. This type of pain is felt in racket sports and may in certain circumstances be experienced by a climber. It is possible that excessive 'dead hanging' (hanging from a hold for a prolonged period) in a training routine could first lead to this type of fatigue and then, as you break through the pain barrier, to injury.

The mobility of our joints is vital not only to our climbing but also to our everyday life and it is therefore important that we treat them with respect. Listen to their moans and groans and do not push past the pain barrier when it comes from the joint region.

LEVERS AND MOTION

The bones and joints form a very complicated system of anatomical levers which allow an almost infinite number of movements to be made. Understanding a little about the biomechanics of climbing should help you make the best of your abilities.

1.   A *lever* is a solid bar which will rotate around a pivot or fulcrum, when an effort is applied. This will move the load on the lever.
2.   The *load* is your weight.

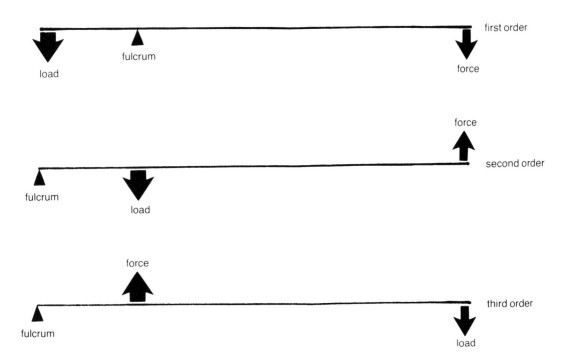

Fig 2 Levers.

3. The *effort* is the muscular contraction to move your weight.

4. The *fulcrum* is the joint about which the movement occurs or the point of contact with the rock.

There are three types of levers. A *first order lever* is one where the fulcrum is between the effort and the load. For example, when standing on a small hold, your Achilles tendon working at the ankle produces a first order lever. With this lever, a small movement of the effort will produce a large movement of the load but the effort must be great.

A *second order lever* has the load between the fulcrum and the effort. For example, if you are hanging on the lip of an overhang about to pull up, then by putting your feet on the rock you produce a second order lever system (this assumes no effort from your legs, which in practice will help as

well). Here the large movement of a small effort moves a large load a small distance, and the effort is noticeably less than if you let your feet swing free, in which case you will be relying upon the third order lever system of your biceps.

A *third order lever* applies the effort between the fulcrum and the load, for example, the biceps acting during a pull-up. Here the effort must be greater than the load, moving through a short distance to move the load through a large distance.

An objective assessment of your ability to move efficiently will point to the areas needing improvement. A balance of strength, speed and flexibility will give the most economical movements and greater choice of movements. Brute force can sometimes compensate for lack of flexibility; similarly, extreme reach can overcome lack of strength. Both situations are far from ideal, however, as the body is put into a mechanically inefficient

13

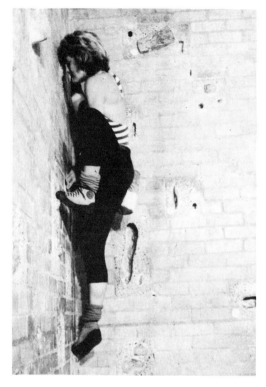 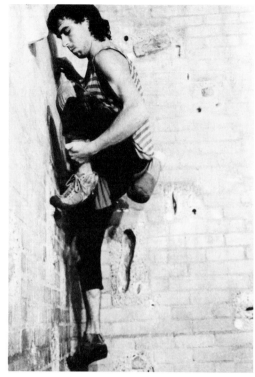

Fig 3 The value of flexibility; Anna is able to keep closer to the wall and does not need to pull her leg up with her hand as Ray does.

situation. A fully extended muscle is at its weakest and has more power in the mid-range of its movement because of the mechanics and physiology involved – it is the ability to apply and co-ordinate whatever strength you may have in the most efficient manner to produce the required movement which is one of the main skills of climbing. You may be able to do a great number of bench presses but unless you have the skill to apply that strength you will not be able to climb well.

MUSCLES

The muscle type that we are primarily interested in is known as *voluntary* or *skeletal* muscle. It is composed of thousands of minute fibres which are bound together by connective tissue to form fasciculi which in turn are bound together to form the muscle itself. It has been recognised for some time that there are different types of voluntary muscle fibres.

Red fibres, known as *slow twitch* or type 1, fibres are capable of a sustained work output. The pale fibres on the other hand seem to depend upon the stored energy sources within the muscle fibres. They are capable of high energy outputs, but only for short periods, as fatigue occurs as the energy store runs out. These are known as *fast twitch fibres* or type 2B fibres. These two types represent the extremes; intermediates, known as *fast twitch oxidation* or type 2A fibres, can work in either way.

Whatever the type of muscle, it is attached to the bone via a tendon which matches the shape of the muscle. Usually the

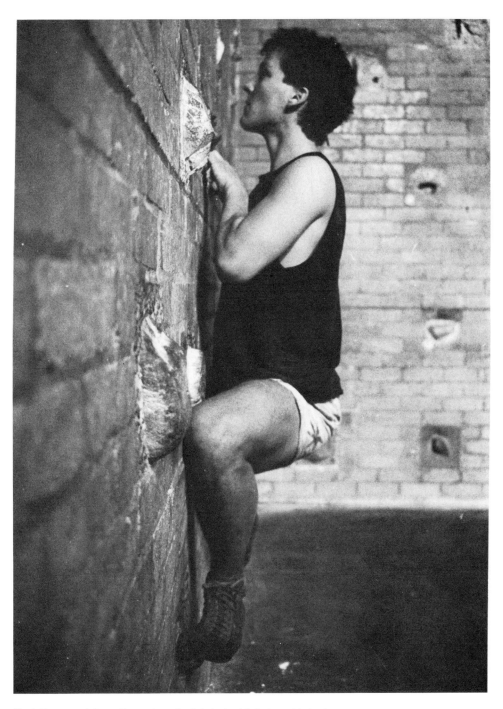

Fig 4 Because Johnny Dawes is so flexible he is able to keep his body
close into the wall and therefore uses less effort.

muscle will run across a joint so that when it contracts it pulls its points of attachment closer thus causing movement about that joint. One end usually remains stationary and has a large area of attachment. This is known as the *origin* of the muscle whilst the other end is known as the *insertion*.

So that the body can move, it is necessary to have muscles grouped into pairs where one, *the agonist*, produces the movement and the other, the *antagonist*, allows the limb to return to its original position. In most movements a number of different muscles are involved; the degree of involvement in any one action will depend upon the size of the muscles involved, the force needed and the angle of pull. Taking the action of a pull-up, the major muscles that are involved around the elbow joint, for example, are the *brachialis, biceps* and the *brachio-radialis*. When little effort is needed, for example if the feet are supported, then only the brachialis will be used. As the effort required increases so first the biceps will be used and then the brachio-radialis. When all of these are working to maximum capacity then others such as the *flexor carpi radialis*, the *flexor carpi ulnaris* and other small muscles which span the elbow joint but which are primarily involved in flexion of the wrist, are brought into use. Muscles can therefore be grouped into four categories:

1. Prime movers; the muscles that contribute most to a movement.
2. Assistant movers; those which, because of their size or angle of pull can only assist in a movement.
3. Stabilisers; these stabilise one end of the muscle so that a joint can move through its full range.
4. Neutralisers; often there can be unwanted secondary movements as a result of a muscle contracting, and these are neutralised by this group. For example, the *pronator quadratus* counteracts the unwanted twisting of the forearm that occurs when the biceps is used.

Muscles contract in a number of different ways. In our pull-up example the muscle shortens and thickens and there is movement of the joint; this is known as a *concentric contraction*. If you now lower yourself down slowly in control then the muscles undergo an *eccentric contraction*, the muscle lengthening under tension. If you lock off at the top of a pull-up then this action is known as an *isometric contraction*. Finally there is one more type of contraction called *isokinetic contraction*. When a muscle group contracts it does not maintain a maximum effort throughout the whole movement (this is because of a combination of physiological and mechanical factors). Because overload is an essential part of training, various machines were constructed to counteract this problem and make the muscle work continually at the same effort throughout a movement. This type of isokinetic contraction does not occur naturally but is very effective as a means of training.

Analysing a muscle action can be very useful as you will then be able to condition that particular group appropriately. This does not need to be very difficult as you need only establish which are the major groups involved – though it can be useful to work out which stabilisers and neutralisers are being used. Start by identifying the joint systems that are employed and then look at the table of muscles in Appendix II to see which muscle groups are involved.

INJURIES

Many top climbers world-wide are now suffering a number of debilitating injuries, the causes of which range from poor training and over-training to just too much climbing. The exact causes are difficult to ascertain until further research has taken place, and what we have written here is not designed to replace a visit to the doctor. On the contrary, we hope that by reading this you will be more inclined to seek medical advice sooner.

One of the major injuries experienced is *peritendinitis*. This is an inflammation of the membrane surrounding the tendon and will occur when the tendon is overloaded or over-used. Because of the varied nature of climbing there are many tendons that can be damaged, though those in the forearms and hands seem to be particularly susceptible. Warming up increases the elastic properties of the muscle tendon unit, therefore it follows that if you do not warm up correctly to a climbing or training session then you are more likely to suffer an injury. If damage does occur then it is repaired by scar tissue, but this tissue is bulky and weak, and the weakness means that it is susceptible to further injury – it is very easy to enter a cycle of injury and re-injury unless you take swift and effective action.

Your first task then is to decide whether or not you are suffering from peritendinitis. Usually you will notice a dull ache, particularly during a muscle contraction and after a hard climb or training session. You can check whether this is likely to be peritendinitis by warming the affected area by doing whatever normally causes pain, and then stretching the limb concerned fully (this may involve more than one joint in which case stretch both joints at either end of the site of injury). Some pain at this point would suggest peritendinitis. With the help of a friend work the suspect limb through its full range of movement and again some pain may be felt. Finally press your thumb into the site of injury, with the limb resting in a comfortable position. Again pain will be felt if it is peritendinitis (the major exception to this is for injuries to the shoulder which are very difficult to diagnose). It must be stressed that if you suspect such an injury you should seek medical advice at the first opportunity and you should rest the injured limb straight away.

If the pain has occurred in the last couple of days and is not too severe then apply some ice to the site and stop training for a week or more. To continue, and to work through the pain barrier is to invite further injury. Isometric exercises are useful because they do not cause the injured tendon to be irritated by joint movement. Pain that has been there for longer periods must be treated by a programme of procedures and the degree of injury can be classified as acute (moderate to severe pain that has been there from two days to four weeks) or chronic (anything that has been there for more than four weeks).

With acute peritendinitis, the first problem is to control the inflammation – this is best done with the use of ice or a cold pack. Massage the site for about five minutes with ice (slightly longer if you are using a cold pack) making sure that you keep the ice moving to prevent frostbite; if numbness occurs before the five minutes are up then stop. The next stage is to apply some local compression for about twenty minutes using an appropriate bandage. Repeating this alternately for the first ten hours after an injury has proved to be most effective. The limb will benefit from being elevated throughout this procedure.

For chronic peritendinitis, the above procedures should be tried, and you should also begin to stretch the injured muscle and tendons, though only slight pain should be felt. The injury should be taped or braced and you should continue to strengthen uninjured muscle so that the compensatory capabilities are improved.

Effective taping is a highly skilled job and if done badly could cause further problems, so it is best to get a physiotherapist to show you how first. Taping works by constraining the full muscle expansion and thereby reducing the overload forces. A reduction of about five per cent is normally achieved and this will not affect performance though the small amount involved becomes significant over countless repetitions that occur when you are climbing or training. You should use two-inch non-stretch tape and it should only be wrapped around the main bulk of the muscle so that it remains comfortable. The tape should only feel tense when the muscle itself is tensed fully.

Finally, there is one more technique

called *transverse friction* that can be used in promoting recovery in both of the above cases. The scar tissue that forms after an injury is a disorganised network of tissues compared to the parallel tissues of a healthy tendon. By applying friction perpendicular to the injured tissue it is possible to break up the scar tissue that has not remodelled itself in the normal direction and this in turn should help to maintain the mobility of the tendon. During the first week of injury it seems to aggravate the injury and should therefore be avoided but in subsequent weeks it can be applied lightly, though if any pain is felt it must be stopped. Usually it is best to treat the tendon in a neutral position, neither stretched nor tensed, and the area to be treated is the exact spot of most pain. Use the thumbs or middle fingers and move the skin above the site of injury at a rate of two cycles per second. After two minutes the tenderness should have subsided and the pressure can be increased for a further three minutes (a total of five minutes should be the maximum period of treatment to start with, though you can work up to ten minutes within ten days). Increase the depth of pressure as much as can be tolerated, though you should never experience pain. There should be a maximum of ten treatments which should take place every other day. If you have skin problems or difficulties with your circulation then do not use this technique.

ENERGY SYSTEMS

The body has three different energy systems. One of them is *aerobic*, that is it uses oxygen, and the other two are *anaerobic* and do not use oxygen. The first of these systems to be used is the start-up system known as the *phosphocreatine* or *alactic* system which combines with a substance called ADP within the muscle cell to produce energy. This stored energy has no by-products and lasts for anything between 10 and 20 seconds depending upon the intensity of the work, and with appropriate training the phospho-creatine level in the body can be raised by up to 200 per cent and possibly even higher.

The main anaerobic system however is the lactic energy system and without going into great detail about the complex chemical exchanges that take place, energy is produced and a by-product, lactic acid results. The energy produced by this system can last up to 2 minutes but then the lactic acid build-up produces fatigue in the muscles.

The final system to consider is the aerobic system which utilises oxygen to liberate energy from the muscle fuels. The energy provided by this system has no detrimental by-products and provided there is an adequate supply of oxygen will last indefinitely.

The relationship between these systems is very important because it will dictate how we adapt our endurance training to suit our needs. All three systems work alongside each other and are inextricably linked together, but it is often useful for the purposes of designing training programmes to examine them separately even though this involves a gross over-simplification of what is actually happening. Looking first at the order in which our body tends to employ the three systems, it is important to realise that the muscle (and remember that it is the ability of the muscle to perform work with which we are concerned) will normally bring in the anaerobic cycles only to supplement the aerobic mechanisms when they are fully stretched.

Imagine you are about to start a climb, a steep climb that will be demanding straight away. The muscle cells hold very little in the way of stored oxygen, therefore, as you start the pitch, the energy will have to come from the anaerobic system since at this moment the aerobic system cannot cope. The lactic system takes a short while to get into gear (as the chemical chain starts to operate) so it is the alactic system that provides the initial source of energy – it is the start-up system. By the time the supply of phosphocreatine runs out, the lactic system should have reached full flow and it will take over.

During this period an oxygen debt will have built up and until it is cleared (usually within a few minutes) the exercise will feel harder. Once a steady state is reached and you get second wind the aerobic system will have taken over (this is a good argument for warming up correctly as it is undesirable to experience your second wind actually on the climb). If the aerobic system cannot cope then the others will be brought into play again. For example, if the climb suddenly steepens, putting more demands on the muscles, the aerobic system may not be able to supply enough energy, and the anaerobic system is then employed. If the steep bit is short and you are then able to rest, you will return to working aerobically and feel none the worse for it (relatively speaking). If, however, the steep section is long and sustained, the muscles will continue to work anaerobically, the alactic cycle rapidly running out of supplies thus causing the lactic system to take on the work-load. It is this system that produces lactic acid and a build-up of this causes the all too familiar 'pumped' sensation. If we cannot relieve this fatigue then eventually we will run out of strength and fall off.

It follows from this scenario that the more efficient our aerobic system is the better, since this will put off the employment of the anaerobic cycle with its penalties. Your first priority should therefore be to raise your anaerobic threshold, the point at which you employ this system. Having done that you can then work upon your anaerobic endurance, improving your reserves of phosphocreatine and improving the mechanisms of producing and clearing lactic acid. The exact balance of this plan will depend upon two basic factors: your physical make-up and your style of climbing (the two may indeed be inextricably linked together).

As we have already pointed out there are three different types of muscle fibres, type 1, type 2A and type 2B. Type 1 works aerobically, type 2A can work either way and type 2B will work anaerobically. The muscle will always tend to employ the different types in the same order, first type 1 then type 2A and finally as the work-load or intensity is increased still further, type 2B. We all have a mixture of these fibres but it follows that climbers with a high proportion of type 1 fibres will have a more efficient aerobic system and vice-versa for those high in type 2B fibres. The former will have to work on their anaerobic endurance and the latter their aerobic.

Your climbing style may be affected by your body make-up but many other factors, not least of which will be your mental approach, will also be important. If, however, you climb in a steady plodding way and rapidly tire on steep hard sections then perhaps you should be looking to build up your anaerobic capabilities; whereas if you can cope with short intense pitches but run out of steam on the longer more sustained routes, concentrating on your aerobic training in order to raise your anaerobic threshold might be beneficial. It is difficult without laboratory testing facilities to be exact, but by looking hard at your climbing style and perhaps at how you perform in other sports (sprinters have a predominance of type 2B fibres and marathon runners of type 1) you should be able to reach some reasonable conclusions and be able to adapt your programmes appropriately.

NUTRITION

With the building of the perfect climbing machine it would seem common sense to fuel it with the best fuel. Good nutrition is not difficult to organise or to find out about and it need not be expensive. A well-balanced diet, with carbohydrate, protein, some fat, minerals and vitamins, will build strong bones and muscles and will also enable all the chemical processes necessary in energy production to take place. There is no need to buy food supplements or diet packs providing you can eat a balanced diet.

Most climbers realise that extra weight is

a burden they can well do without and some go to extraordinary lengths to get rid of it. Most people seem to have a metabolic rate which keeps their weight within certain limits, even though some may eat much more or much less than others. You can increase your metabolic rate with aerobic exercise and reduce your body fat content. You can build muscle with exercise, so that your weight may increase but your fat:lean ratio will decrease. Fresh fruit and vegetables, whole grain products, dairy products fish and lean meat will provide all the dietary requirements. Junk foods, being for the most part just that, are best avoided; you owe yourself better than that. Sugar does not have to be eaten for energy, as that comes from breaking down carbohydrates, which if eaten in the form of whole grain (rice, bread, pasta), potatoes and other vegetables, also provides vitamins and minerals.

Diets are fashionable and it is easy to become disillusioned with the many varying and often contrasting ideas around, so eat sensibly and if you do embark upon any special diet record your progress in exactly the same way as you would with your other training programmes so that you can see if it is having the desired effect.

DRUGS

Many climbers have in the past experimented with drugs of one sort or another to aid them to a better performance. Most of the drugs used are not only illegal but interfere with the body's processes and hence your ability to listen to its signals; the result is invariably injury and ill health. Do not be tempted by the apparent attractions of using them, the gains are always short-lived and the costs, in terms of your health, are just too high.

2　The Basics of Training

In this section we will be looking at the areas of the body that we can train and the physiological processes that will occur during such training. The greater the understanding of this part of the book the easier it will be to adapt training programmes to your own needs and situation.

TERMINOLOGY

There are a number of concepts that are basic to all forms of training and it is necessary to understand these in order to gain the full benefit from your efforts. It is also necessary to clarify some simple terminology that will enable you to interpret later passages more easily.

Overload

In order that physiological changes can occur, it is necessary to stress the body systems above a certain level, making it work harder than normal. The amount of overload is known as the *intensity*. As your programme advances and your body adapts it will be necessary to increase the work-load in order to continue to overload the body's systems. This is known as *progressive overloading*.

Rests

During a training session, as the work is being undertaken the body's resources are being depleted. After the workout the body will go through a recovery period which is followed by a period of enhancement and it is at this moment that you should train again. If you leave it until after the enhancement period, you will merely be maintaining your current level of fitness not improving it; if you train before this period then you will be depleting the body's reserves still further and will effectively be lowering your level of fitness (*see* Fig 79). The rest periods of any programme are as vital as any of the work periods, as it is during these periods that most of the physiological changes that result from your training will take place. To establish the correct intervals, you must keep records of your level of fitness. If it declines, your rest periods are too short; if it stays constant, they are too long.

Reversibility

The effects of all forms of training are reversible if the training is infrequent or the intensity insufficient.

Specificity

The effects of your training are specific to the type of training you undertake. This applies not only to the energy systems being employed, but also to the individual muscles being used and even to the range and type of movement that they use during the activity for which you are training. It follows therefore that you will have to evaluate your own needs carefully in order to get the most effect from your training.

Monitoring

The effect of your training should be monitored at frequent intervals for several reasons:

1.　To make sure that the programme you have followed is having the desired effect.
2.　It will help to motivate you.
3.　So that you may make decisions about when to alter a programme, to increase its intensity or to change it in order to work a different energy system, for example.

In the text we have offered a number of ways of monitoring your progress, none of which require special equipment. If you have access to specially designed equipment then take the opportunity to use it and record your findings, such research will be most helpful in planning future training programmes.

It is important that, whatever system you use to record your progress, you make comparisons with your own previous performance and not that of others. This is because they are normally meaningless when out of context and the effect of comparing your performance with others in this way is usually detrimental to motivation.

Adaptability

A flexible approach in a programme is essential to allow for fluctuations in your health and individual differences and requirements.

Repetitions

Commonly called reps, these are the number of times an exercise is repeated without stopping. An important idea to understand is what is known as the *repetition maximum* or RM. This is the maximum load a muscle group can lift a predetermined number of times before it gets tired. A *set* is a specific number of repetitions and *resistance* is the load that a muscle group is required to move.

ENDURANCE TRAINING

Endurance can mean many things to many people – the ability to do a sequence of hard moves on a rock climb, to survive the rigours of a Himalayan storm, or even just lasting an Alpine hut walk!

As we have seen there are basically two energy systems used by the body, the aerobic system, which uses oxygen (O_2), and the anaerobic system which operates when there is insufficient oxygen to meet demands. It is therefore desirable to improve your capacity for aerobic work first, off-setting the moment when the anaerobic system might be employed. This is important because it is the anaerobic system that produces by-products which contribute to fatigue.

The O_2 must be transported efficiently to the muscle by the cardio-respiratory system, and used effectively by the muscle. About 10 litres of air per minute are breathed when the body is at rest and this can be raised to 150 litres per minute during hard work. The most that can be breathed through the nose is about 50 litres per minute, after which mouth breathing becomes a necessity. Generally it is much more efficient to take large breaths than short, quick ones which will tax the respiratory muscles more and not allow enough time for the blood to absorb the O_2. It follows that if you are trying to rest then it would be better to take deep breaths using the stomach muscles. Concentrate on breathing out, as control of this phase will help you control the whole respiratory cycle. Using the stomach muscles may help your already over-taxed shoulder and chest muscles relax more – every little helps!

Training affects the lungs very little; what does change, however, is the mechanism for transporting the O_2, the heart and the blood. A resting heart pumps about 5 litres per minute whereas a trained one during activity can pump up to 30 or more litres per minute. This increase is achieved in two ways. Firstly, the pulse rate rises to a maximum which is age dependent (on average it is 220 minus your age) and is unaffected by training. Secondly, the stroke volume, which is affected by training, will increase. At very high heart rates, 90–95 per cent of maximum, the heart struggles to fill its chambers, and there is just insufficient time for the blood to flow in. It is, therefore, necessary to work the heart at a percentage of its maximum, the training zone, (any more will be ineffective at training the aerobic

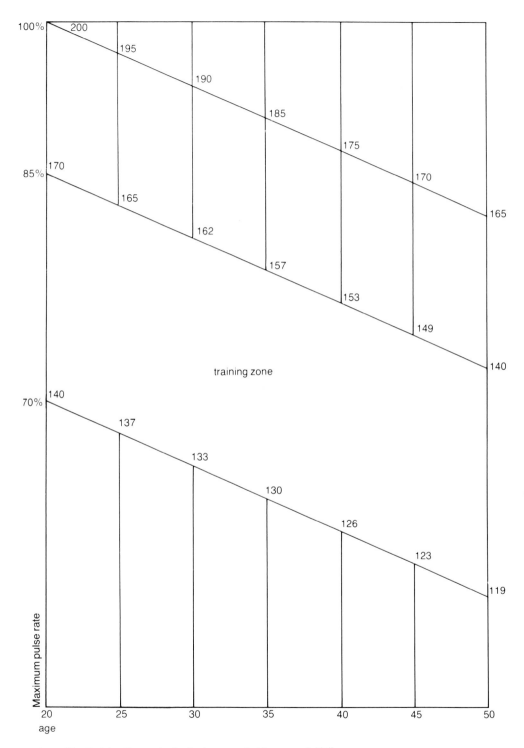

Fig 5 The Training Zone; aim for the lower end of the range initially.

system) and you can work this out from Fig 5. This filling problem can cause faintness at the end of a strenuous workout but should not be anything to worry about. It should go if you warm down slowly, if not, consult your doctor.

Training also promotes the growth of capillaries, and can actually increase the volume of blood by up to 50 per cent. Strangely, more plasma is produced than red O^2-absorbing cells, resulting in a condition known as *sports anaemia*. This may have implications for the high altitude climber and the rate at which one acclimatises. After acclimatisation the blood is thicker, by virtue of the increased number of red cells, thus causing the heart to work harder. Dehydration, which in turn lowers the output of the heart, is therefore more significant at altitude.

The whole purpose of aerobic training is to get more O^2 to the muscles, and recent research has confirmed that the training should be specific. A swimmer gets less improvement in aerobic performance from using running as a training medium compared to using swimming for example. It follows that Alpinists may want to concentrate on their legs whereas rock climbers will want to bias their programme towards their upper body. This is known as specifying.

Before embarking upon a scheme, you should set yourself goals and record your progress towards them. Make your goal-setting appropriate. For example, an increase of 10 per cent over the first month should be attainable, but it is far better to go for a 1 per cent increase at each of the 10 sessions (average 3 sessions a week), as it will seem less daunting. Training yourself to do this will be as hard as the work itself! Measuring your progress is not easy but it is important and should only be done in a way that compares your current level of fitness against your own previous level not against others. A study by Buske and Borg has shown that people are very accurate at assessing the level of difficulty of a training session. If we divide the level of difficulty into say 20

stages, 0 is no effort and 20 means you think you are going to die (you should never be able to reach 20). If it normally takes an effort of 18 to achieve your programme and you start to be able to do it with an effort of only 10 or 11, then you know you are making progress. This method can be very accurate, but remember the fitter you are the harder it becomes to achieve any improvement.

A similar method is to record your pulse rate immediately after a specific exercise, this exercise remaining the same throughout your training, and then record how long it takes for your pulse to return to its resting rate. The shorter the period the fitter you are becoming.

The optimum length for a training session is about 30 minutes (no less) with a warm-up and warm-down period either side. Three sessions a week would appear to be the most advantageous frequency. There are a number of forms of training you can use and we believe that variety is the key to maintaining motivation. Whichever medium you employ it is very important to warm up and down correctly and we suggest that you also stretch before and after activity.

Running

As it is very difficult for any other muscle group, except the legs, to make sufficient demands on the cardio-respiratory system running is an ideal form of exercise. It also trims the muscles down reducing lower body weight positively; therefore we suggest that this medium be your starting point. The biggest improvements will be made during the first 4–8 weeks of your programme. It is the length of time (ideally, 30 minutes) that your heart rate is within the training zone that is important not the mileage covered, although as you will see a variety of effects can be achieved by varying speed and distance. Aim to reach the lower end of the training zone initially, reaching the higher limits in the 6th to 8th week. If you increase the effort too quickly then you will end up working anaerobically, the lactic acid will build up, muscle fatigue will result and your attempts to improve your cardio-respiratory system will be lost. It is easy to judge your progress with running because you can record your time over a set distance. Because a rock-climber's O^2 uptake will vary throughout a climb it will be advisable after about the 4th week to add some variations to the run to simulate this and this can be achieved in several ways.

Interval running consists of running specified distances in a given time with a rest between. This is very good for the lower body, and if structured correctly can be made to work either the aerobic system or the anaerobic system. It is an extremely efficient method of training the athlete's ability to recover from work if the bursts are at maximal effort. It could be said, however, that it is a method most suited to the runner and has limited use for the climber.

Of perhaps more relevance to the climber is a popular technique know as fartlek. Some running coaches recommend that you vary your speed according to how your body feels, for example short fast sections interspersed with slower periods, and others say you should structure it carefully in a well-planned fashion to create overload situations with suitable rest periods. Which method you choose may depend upon the type of terrain in which you are training. If the terrain is hilly then you can use the naturally occuring changes of rhythm but if it is flat you will have to introduce your own variations. Start with a warming up jog of say five minutes. Follow this by a faster-paced section but not flat out; take a short resting section and follow this by a fast pace interspersed with short sections at your maximum pace. Rest again and then repeat it over again, finally slowing down and repeating the initial pattern in reverse. The exact length of each section will depend upon your own level of fitness, and you will have to gauge this by how you feel. It is, despite its *ad hoc* nature, a very effective medium. The short burst of sprinting forces you to employ the anaerobic system, the oxygen debt that

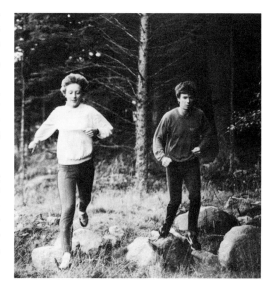

Fig 6 A form of fartlek circuit; Anita and Steve use a simple circuit, starting with a run.

results demands repayment and this situation stimulates improvements in your ability to take up oxygen and to recover. It is designed to allow the athlete to recover from short bursts of activity which are followed by more, less intense, periods of work and as such is ideally suited to the climber's situation. Taking this idea further and specialising more closely, you could insert into your run 2 to 3 minute periods of push-ups, pull-ups, and dips (Figs 6, 7 and 8). Many people have created circuits within areas of woodland which facilitate this form of training.

Long, slow, distance training is used by many and here the emphasis is on a long-sustained, low-intensity effort. This type of exercise enhances fat metabolism and therefore offers some promise of weight control. The training of the fat metabolism in this way may help the Alpinist to use fat more efficiently, thus preserving the carbohydrates. It is this painful switch to fat that has to occur when the carbohydrate runs out that is the cause of the 'wall' in marathon runners. Running constantly at a faster pace (closer to your maximum pace over a set distance) on the other hand, will develop the

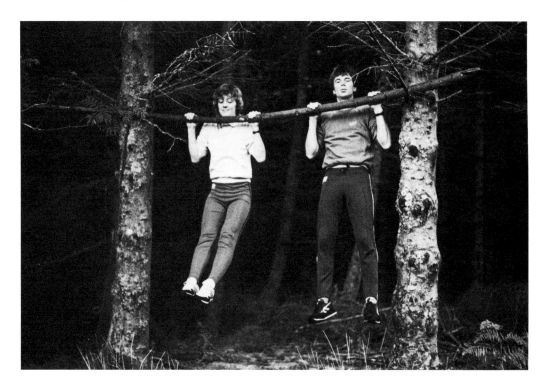

Fig 7 A pull-ups station.

carbohydrate aerobic pathways. Variety would appear to be the key word for the climber using running as a training medium – you do not want to stereotype yourself by sticking to only one method.

Running badly can do more harm than good, so it is important to invest in a good pair of appropriate running shoes, warm up and down correctly and ideally run on grass rather than roads. Most good sports shops should be able to give you good advice about the type of shoe to consider.

In a recent study (1987), Dr Rick Turner of Birmingham University demonstrated that cardio-vascular fitness has a direct bearing on our ability to cope with stress. Normally, the heart works at a rate appropriate to the physical demands put on it. Under stressful situations, people with a high level of cardio-vascular fitness experienced a smaller increase in heart rate than those who were less fit. If the physical demands of climbing

are already causing your heart rate to increase, then it is of benefit to know that the psychological stresses of the route can be coped with, without raising it too much more.

Circuit Training

The beauty of this medium is that it can be set up almost anywhere, with a little imagination, and it is also easy to specify by emphasising those exercises that work the particular muscle groups relevant to you. Examples of actual exercises can be found later in the book; here we will concern ourselves with the principles of circuit training.

Introduce it after about four weeks of running if you are starting a programme. There are a variety of ways in which you can plan your circuits, though all of them should contain between 8 and 15 different stations.

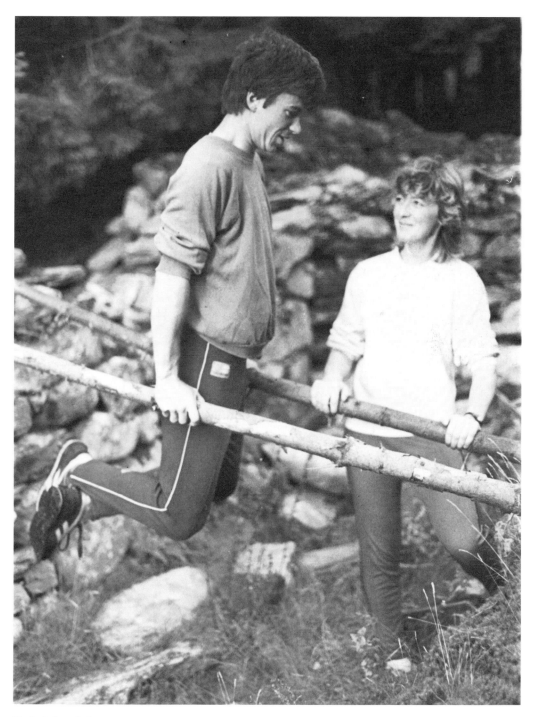

Fig 8 A dips station.

There may be a number of different exercises possible at any one station. Be careful to avoid having the same muscle groups worked on at adjacent stations. When you arrive at a station you can do a number of predetermined repetitions (sufficient to cause noticeable fatigue) and then try to complete the whole circuit within a given time span. Alternatively, you can complete the greatest number of circuits within that time span, or you can work for a set period at each station making sure that you allow enough time to cause fatigue. Another alternative is to find out the maximum number of repetitions you can do for each exercise (it should number at least fifteen in order to work the aerobic system) and then perform each circuit according to the following:

1st circuit at ½ maximum repetitions
2nd circuit at ¾ maximum repetitions
3rd circuit at maximum repetitions

No rest should be taken between any stations, but a rest is appropriate between circuits. These rest periods are very important as the physiological processes taking place during them are as relevant as those that occur during the work periods.

The variations, as you can appreciate, are endless. Working with a partner can help in many ways in that they can help to motivate you and they can be a substitute for apparatus if you do not have a gym in which to train. Once you have done the circuits for a while you may like to introduce some skills training into the routine. Performing skilful tasks under the stress created by a strenuous circuit can be very valuable. For example, at the top of a rope climb, clip a karabiner into a preplaced prussik loop attached to the rope; or when you are doing lock-offs clip a karabiner to a sling whilst locked off. The wall can be used effectively at this stage by introducing difficult technical problems within the structure of your circuit.

Weights

Again, specific exercises are detailed later. The addition of weights to the above circuits will increase the number of options open to you, though if you are under 16 years of age you should not use them without the supervision of a qualified coach – you can do serious damage to yourself at this age because your body is still growing. If you have access to a multi-gym, then it is easy to design a circuit around its stations. Whatever type of weights you use it is the number of repetitions that you use that is important. You should be working with a weight that allows you to do between 15 and 20 repetitions rapidly and this usually works out to be about 70 per cent of the maximum weight you can move. The number of reps can be increased when you are fitter, to improve the local muscular endurance of a particular muscle group. Before using weights to help with your endurance training be sure to read the section devoted to specific exercises.

Swimming

If you want to add some variety to your programme, then swimming may be useful. Treat it as though you were running and add arms or legs only sections in order to specify.

Canoeing and Rowing

We think the potential for the rock climber if you have access to this medium could be very good. It certainly works the upper body and furthermore it is possible to work these muscle groups aerobically – although the restricted action may prove to be too specific to these sports and therefore the carry-over to climbing may be limited.

Cycling

This medium has relatively little value to the rock climber but could be good for the Alpinist as it is an excellent medium for working the cardio-respiratory system and the legs.

The Wall/Bouldering

On many walls and boulders it is difficult to work the body aerobically. Even if the wall's design allowed it, other users often get in the way of a proper routine. If, however, you are lucky enough to have access to a wall or boulders on which it is possible to train aerobically then they have to be one of the best mediums to use. It may be possible to introduce the wall or a boulder as a station into a circuit or even to work on a number of circuits on them. A particular sequence of moves may stress one muscle group and another sequence a different set. Traverse in both directions and go up and down – and even rotary problems can be worked out. By following the principles outlined above and with a degree of ingenuity it is possible to work out some interesting circuits, but whatever use you do make of it, be sure it is training your body in the way you want it to – there may at this stage of your overall programme be a better medium.

For the reasons explained earlier we suggest that you spend the first couple of months of your programme building up your aerobic fitness and only then should you move on to developing your anaerobic endurance and strengthening certain muscle groups.

ANAEROBIC ENDURANCE

Anaerobic endurance is short term and is normally brought into play when the aerobic system can no longer cope. This usually occurs in three situations.

1. At the beginning of a climb or on the walk in, before the aerobic system has got going a small oxygen debt builds up. The deficit is quickly repaid and in any case only happens during the first 30 seconds or so. While you are repaying this deficit however you will feel as though the work is harder.

2. In very explosive actions such as 'dynos' which last only for a second or two, the aerobic system does not have the time to act.
3. Any intense burst of climbing lasting from about 10 seconds to up to 2 minutes could be almost completely anaerobic. This will include most of the crux moves on many climbs but providing you are flexible and have a well-developed aerobic system it should be only these cruxes where this system is employed.

Once you have trained your aerobic system it may be desirable to work upon your anaerobic endurance specifically. If you think you are an endurance climber (high in type 1 muscle fibres) then you should concentrate on lactate production and if you are an explosive type of climber (high in type 2 muscle fibres) then your training should be biased towards the removal of lactate. The latter is achieved by programming the work intervals to be long (a minute or even longer) and the rest intervals to be short (about 30 seconds), whereas in the former it is necessary to keep the work interval short (30 – 40 seconds) and the rest period long (3–5 minutes).

The rest intervals in anaerobic training are vital. They allow time for the clearance of lactic acid, which takes place in two stages, firstly into the blood and secondly out of the blood. The clearance of the lactic acid from the muscle into the blood is probably the most important phase to the climber, who, like the gymnast, is generally using smaller muscle groups at a time. When a muscle stops working, the flow of blood drops off within about 20 seconds and this will tend to lock up the lactic acid. It follows therefore that a continuation of the work at a lower level will maintain a good blood flow and allow a more efficient clearance of the fatigue-causing lactic acid. The level of activity seems to vary according to the muscle groups being employed but until further laboratory testing has occurred specific to the needs of the climber you will have to experiment yourself in order to discover just how hard to work during these active rest periods in order to promote maximum recovery in the shortest possible time.

As was noted earlier, anaerobic endurance makes use of two energy systems, the phosphagen system and the lactic system, each of which can be trained specifically.

Phosphagen System

Exercise must be performed at a maximum, the *duration* of the exercise should be not less than 5, and no more than 20 seconds, and the overall *volume* (total time of session) should last for about 6–8 minutes. It is essential that this type of training is performed at maximum intensity and in order to maintain the quality of work a ratio of 5:1 or 6:1 of rest to work should be allowed between repetitions and an active recovery period of about 5–10 minutes between sets is necessary.

Lactic Energy System

With the provisos mentioned earlier, the *intensity* of the exercise should be in the region of 90 per cent of your maximum for any given exercise. Work intervals should be of about 40 – 60 seconds in length and never longer than 2 minutes as you will then be taxing the aerobic system. The overall volume can be anywhere between 10 and 20 minutes. Start with a work:rest ratio of 1:2 and gradually change it to 1:1 and finally to 2:1 with about 10 minutes of active resting between sets.

STRENGTH

Strength is the maximum force which a muscle or group of muscles can exert against a resistance. If you cannot do a pull-up or a one arm pull-up then it is the strength of the muscle groups involved in this movement that need to be built up. If, however, you can do a pull-up but want to be able to do more without tiring then it will be the endurance of that group that will have to be worked upon.

In order to develop the strength of a particular muscle it is necessary to overload that muscle and it is generally accepted that the best way in which to do this is to work with weights. The weight can take several forms: it can be your own body weight or that of a partner; it can be in the form of free weights, for example a barbell or dumbbell; as a machine (either one offering progressive resistance or one offering isokinetic resistance); or it can be an immovable object offering isometric resistance. Which you choose will depend upon the facilities available and the requirements of your programme. Most isokinetic machines for instance will only work on concentric contractions and many climbing moves could involve eccentric contractions. Free weights tend to work the stabilising muscles as well and are therefore good in developing balanced control, and multi-gyms are very safe to use, so all mediums have different pros and cons.

Whichever medium you use there are a number of rules which must be observed in order to reduce the chances of injury.

1. Seek expert advice about how to use a particular piece of equipment (later we will be recommending a number of exercises but you should still get advice about how to use the equipment available to you).
2. Decide exactly what you want to get out of your weight training, the area of fitness you wish to develop and the muscle groups you want to work on.
3. Warm up correctly; stretch before and after a workout.
4. Never lift weights heavier than your programme calls for.
5. Keep a tidy gym and observe its safety rules. More accidents occur from the neglect of this rule than any other.

6. Wear the correct clothing. Keep yourself covered, as wet equipment due to sweat becomes slippery and dangerous.

7. Keep a record so that you can chart your progress.

8. Do not lift heavy weights alone.

9. Do not do weight training before a skills session (climbing wall/bouldering) as the fatigue caused by the weights workout will hamper the acquisition of the skills.

10. Do not train with weights before running, as tired leg muscles will not support the knee and hip joints adequately and injury could result.

11. Do not miss workouts – commitment to your programme is essential.

12. Treat the equipment with respect and be especially careful when handling weights.

13. Start a programme with light weights so that you learn the movements correctly. The quality of the movement is more important than the weight pushed (see section on exercises).

After establishing where and on what you are going to train, you can then begin to work out your strength training programme. The first thing you must do is to learn the movements of each exercise. This should be done with light weights and the photographs will help. If a particular exercise is not shown seek expert advice on how to do it properly. Incorrect movements will not only be more likely to cause injury but may not train the muscles in the most appropriate manner.

Secondly, after warming up properly you should work out what is the maximum weight that you can push on each exercise. To avoid injury work up to this maximum. Your training weights will now be calculated from this maximum: a low load is 35–50 per cent of the maximum; a medium load is 55–60 per cent of the maximum; a high load is 70–100 per cent of the maximum. There are different types of sets that you can use and in this chapter we will illustrate those most appropriate to building up strength.

Single Sets

One set using one muscle group is completed and then you move on to the next muscle group. Additional loading is achieved by doing more than one circuit or by increasing the number of repetitions. You should be working initially with a medium load that you can repeat 10 times; when you can do 15 reps increase the weight so that you are reduced to only being able to do 10 reps again. This is a good system for those new to or just starting weight training.

Progressive Resistance

In this case work out your ten repetition maximum (10 RM), the maximum weight you can lift for ten reps. Do each exercise with a short rest (2 minutes) between sets. The first set should be done at 50 per cent of your 10 RM, the second set at 75 per cent and the third set at 100 per cent. As soon as you can do 13 reps of the last set then a new RM will have to be established.

Pyramids

This is one of the best sets for strength training. Having established your maximum, say 50kg for a particular exercise, you should work your reps out as follows, increasing the load by 5kg each time or by 2.5kg if you are very fit.

Average	Very Fit
9 reps at 30kg	40kg
7 reps at 35kg	42.5kg
5 reps at 40kg	45kg
3 reps at 45kg	47.5kg
1 rep at 50kg	50kg (maximum)

As soon as you can achieve 3 reps of this maximum increase the loading throughout. It is now possible to work the sequence in reverse but this is an advanced routine and should only be attempted well into your programme.

Isometric Training

This involves a muscular contraction against an immovable resistance and tends to see the greatest improvements at the angle at which the joint is worked. The contractions should be held for about six seconds at two-thirds maximum force. Generally, this form of training will have few applications for climbers, though it may be a good way to train for lock-offs (holding a pull-up in the up position). However, because it is so specific and climbing demands such variation we feel that there will usually be a more appropriate form of training.

Plyometrics

These are exercises designed to produce the explosive power needed in jumping activities and they may well have an application at the top of our sport where 'dynos' are used frequently. The principle is that the more a muscle is pre-stretched from its natural length before being contracted, the larger the load that can be moved. This is a similar reaction to the one we find if we stretch an elastic band: the more we stretch it the more powerfully it returns to its original position. In a muscle, however, it is not the magnitude of the stretch that is important but rather the speed of the stretch and this point must be remembered when designing plyometric exercises. This phenomenon appears to be the result of two effects: firstly, as the muscle is stretched, so the stretch receptors cause a powerful contraction to prevent muscle damage due to overstretching; and secondly, it makes use of the elastic nature of the fibres surrounding the muscle.

Great care must be exercised if you are using this principle, as it can severely stress the joints involved. Sufficient strength must be built first – usually it is recommended that the muscle group should be able to cope with moving about 1.5 to 2 times the maximum load of the exercise. For example, a common plyometric exercise is to jump from a box to the ground and rebound immediately – before doing this you should be able to do a full squat with 1.5 to 2 times your own body weight. You will be able to adapt many of your normal exercises into a plyometric routine by introducing this explosive element with a degree of pre-stretching but again be very careful, especially if you are doing them with your upper body, as the stress on your joints can be enormous. Ask yourself if you really do need this type of strength in your climbing repertoire.

Finally, remember that too much strength can be detrimental because as the muscle gets stronger so it creates greater internal pressure, which in turn can reduce the amount of blood getting in, thereby limiting its endurance. It would appear that ideally a muscle group should be able to handle about 3 times the maximum needed by the movements involved, though this calculation needs care otherwise we might assume that it is necessary to do a pull-up with a friend hanging from each leg!

FLEXIBILITY

A flexible body is efficient because it allows the various parts to move through the ranges of movement for which they were designed. Lack of flexibility means less range of movement and a shorter effective range in which the muscles can work. All athletes require a degree of flexibility in order to execute the skills of their chosen sport effectively. It is required in different degrees and body location depending on the specific requirements of that sport, for example, swimmers need flexible shoulders and hurdlers need flexible hips and hamstrings. Alpinists should include flexibility training to complement their overall fitness programme and to prevent injury. Modern hard rock climbing or rock gymnastics requires the same sort of flexibility to that found in gymnasts, in most parts of the body other than perhaps the spine. Some of the

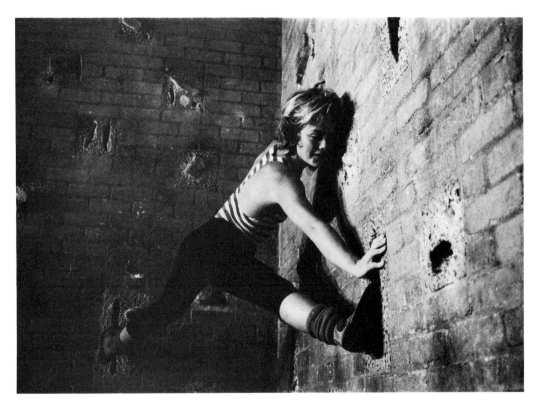

Fig 9 A wide bridge, everybody can appreciate the value of a flexible body in situations like this.

positions attained on modern routes require an extreme range of movement.

The advantages of a good range of movement are many.

1. To provide a wider range for the muscles to work in; more reach; a wider bridge.
2. More movement at the joints lowers the risk of injury when the joint is under stress.
3. To strengthen the muscles, because they can move over a wider range. You cannot strengthen a muscle in a position it cannot get into.
4. To make more efficient use of body strength because of better body positioning relative to holds, and bearing in mind effective use of levers.
5. To make more efficient use of energy

because of less resistance from the muscles that are the antagonists.

Stretching should be an integral part of every training session and fitness programme for several reasons.

1. It prepares muscles and joints for the stresses they will be subjected to during exercise, making them more pliable and less likely to suffer injury.
2. Because of the added range of movement, the muscles can be strengthened over that range.
3. Strengthening exercises shorten and toughen muscle fibres, stretching afterwards helps to correct this.
4. Muscle soreness after hard exercise can be reduced with the right kind of

stretching, immediately afterwards and the next day.

Stretching like strengthening is reversible and so must be considered a permanent part of a fitness programme, so that the benefits are not lost. Stiffness is caused by a number of factors.

1. Bone structure; we cannot alter this.
2. Joint capsules. Bearing in mind that part of the function of these structures is joint stability, great care must be taken. As they are made of soft tissue they can therefore be stretched, but you may then lose some of the integrity of the joint. For example, full squats will stretch the joint capsule in the front of the knee.
3. Muscles, especially large over-developed ones.
4. Tendons.
5. Fat deposits, especially in the trunk/hip area.
6. Results of injury/trauma, or lack of use.

We cannot or do not want to do anything about numbers one and two but we can work upon the others.

Climbers are obviously aware of the advantages of freedom of movement, hence the speed with which they have adopted 'second skins', their lycra tights. This is a quick easy way to get some freedom of movement but working from the inside is more important and everyone can do it.

Stretching exercises fall into two catergories:

1. Those you do before and after a climbing or training session, as preparation and recovery.
2. Those you do specifically to increase your range of movement, much as you would have a session in the weights room or on the climbing wall to increase strength or endurance.

To understand the different ways of lengthening connective tissue and lessening muscle tension, some knowledge of muscle structure and nervous supply is needed. As we have seen, skeletal muscle is made of bundles of fibres which can shorten or be lengthened. These are held together by connective tissue which, at the end of the muscle, becomes continuous with the tendon that crosses the joint before becoming anchored into the bone. In cross section, the tendon is much smaller than the muscle, and transmits the forces produced by the muscle to the bone that is to be moved. Tendon is very tough and not very elastic.

The nervous supply is both sensory and motor thereby monitoring what is happening in the muscle and stimulating a response from the muscle. Normal stretch receptors on the nerve spindles react when the muscle lengthens by signalling the muscle to contract and thus maintain its position *(myotatic reflex)*. This happens all the time to stop you falling over or dropping things for example. A rapid stretch can fire this response, causing a situation where the muscle fibres being lengthened fast and out of control (as in bouncing), will contract, with possible damage being caused. This response is not invoked in slow stretching.

Extreme stretching, to the limits imposed by the elasticity of the muscle, fires a different response. This is from the golgi tendon organ, which is a sensory nerve body in the tendon itself. As previously mentioned, the tendon has far more strain imposed on it per unit of area of its cross section, than the muscle. The golgi body senses extreme tension and responds by inhibiting the muscle from contracting, allowing it to lengthen and thus avoiding tearing (Matthews & Fox). From this we can see that slow stretching is safe and fast stretching, which includes limb swinging and bouncing, is not to be recommended.

The active PNF *(proprioceptive neuromuscular facilitation)* method of stretching (Hardy) is used by many coaches in various sports and is based on a physiotherapy method of treating tissues shortened by injury or after surgery. It helps gains in flexibility to be made at a faster rate than slow stretching or fast stretching, but must be used with great care and taught under supervision. It would be advisable to find someone running a class which employs PNF if you want to learn it. Various methods of PNF have been employed (Holt et al, Tanigawa, Cornelius and Hinson), but the active PNF method seems to have some advantages.

This example shows how PNF would work on hamstrings (a particularly neglected muscle group in many climbers). The person to be stretched would first warm up, keep warm clothing on and lie flat with the leg to be stretched up off the floor in the position of maximum hip flexion. The helper kneels and simply holds the leg in that position, where discomfort but not pain is felt behind the knee. The subject presses hard against the helper with the leg, trying to push it to the floor and breathing naturally as he does so. The helper resists for a count of 6 seconds, then both relax slowly and the subject uses the thigh muscles to pull the leg closer in to the body, thus elongating the hamstrings. The hamstrings are contracting but not altering length (isometric contraction) for a maximum effort up to 6 seconds. After the relaxation, which varies in length with different people, the subject ought to be able to flex at the hip joint (concentric contraction of the quadriceps) to a closer angle with the body than before. The gain may be minimal, or startlingly large, again this depends on different people's responses. There are strict rules for this procedure:

1. Always warm up first.
2. Do this with someone you know, who appreciates the significance and technique.
3. The helper never pushes the limb, merely keeps it in place.
4. Always count to six, relax slowly then move the limb into the new position.

In PNF the slow stretch to maximum extension overcomes the myotatic stretch reflex of the muscle stretch receptors. The iso-metric contraction of the muscle to be stretched stimulates the golgi tendon organ as it stretches the tendon, and the muscle relaxes and lengthens even more. The muscle moving the limb to the new position has a strength gain as it actively stretches the other muscle to its new longer length. You can do this on yourself by assuming a position of maximum extension, using the floor or wall to keep the limb in place and press hard against it in the same way you would against a partner.

From this it should be obvious that rapid stretching is to be avoided, slow stretching is fine and PNF is the best for increasing your mobility. Stretching should be done before and after each session in the weights room, on the climbing wall, or on the rock. The preparatory session is the most important of these two. First warm up, with skipping, jumps and so on. Gentle movement of all the joints, using a logical progression from the neck down, stimulates a flow of lubricating fluid within the joints. Take each joint carefully to a position of maximum stretch, not as far as feeling pain, but a definite limit of movement. Move the limb carefully through its full range of movement but do not swing it vigorously out of control. Before weight training ensure that the muscles to be strengthened are properly stretched along with their opposing muscle. This ensures that they can stretch easily without damage, but are not so stiff that they cause an added resistance to the load on the muscle being strengthened.

After training (weights, climbing wall or a route) stretch again, particularly any muscle feeling pumped up, giving particular attention to fingers and forearms. This helps to reduce shortening of the muscle, and to alleviate muscle soreness. This procedure can also be used the next day if soreness persists. Hold the position of maximum stretch for 2 minutes followed by 1 minute of rest. Repeat 3 times. This is *not* recommended for damaged muscles (W.Wright et al.). Stiffness is at its worst first thing in the morning and last thing at night and so more care or time should be given to stretching at those times.

In a session set aside specifically to work on flexibility your approach should be somewhat different. This should last at least 30 minutes and be repeated twice or even three times a week. The following procedure should be followed:

1. Raise your body temperature to make the muscles more extensible. This need not be a vigorous business. Indeed it seems that there are more gains to be made in flexibility after a passive warm up than an active one. The best way to do this is to have a warm bath until you are relaxed, then a short (1 minute) cool shower to drive the warm blood in the skin deep into the muscles (Hardy).

2. Try to feel mentally relaxed as tension is unproductive. Have a comfortable warm place to work in and maybe play some music.

3. Start with moderate, passive exercises first, where the positions are simply held for 30 seconds, alternating muscle groups. Graduate to more difficult exercises, where you really reach into each position at maximum stretch, hold for 20 seconds, reach a little further for another 10 seconds and move ryhthmically and steadily to the next, repeating them three times. After about ten minutes (you will soon learn to recognise when you are ready), you can be quite active in your methods and use PNF if you have a partner. If you are working alone you can adapt the PNF method by using the floor to resist against instead of a partner. Use the positions illustrated later as a guide, but realise that they show the position you are aiming to achieve eventually, not where you start from.

The benefits of stretching are apparent after one session; they are cumulative and much more obvious after several weeks of training. You will find a fairly rewarding gain after 3–4 weeks. This will continue until you achieve a good level of flexibility. Levelling off in the rate of progress is normal and, as we are not looking for the extremes to be seen in gymnastics, the frequency and length of sessions may be reduced with time. Flexibility gains, however, are reversible, so this period of levelling off should be carefully monitored.

You can devise a measuring system to suit you. If you normally do your workout at home, then you can use sticky tape to mark the floor with a line against which you can measure your splits or lunges. If you do your workouts in different places then you can record the extent of movement with a tape measure. Most people, however, are very much aware of the limits to their flexibility and only seem to become unaware if they cease to do their usual sport. Remember it is easier to maintain a level of fitness than to regain it.

3 Exercises

CIRCUIT TRAINING

The following is a series of exercises ideally suited to circuit training though they could also form the start of any strength training programme. We have divided them into three groups, categorised by the major muscle groups that are employed. Which you decide to use will be determined by the facilities available, by the specification you desire and by your particular life-style. The list is by no means exhaustive and your local sports hall specialist should be able to suggest further exercises if you tell them which muscles you want to work. First, warm up with a 5 minute run.

Upper Body

1. *Press ups* Start with your hands beneath your shoulders, getting wider apart as you get fitter (Fig. 10). If these are too difficult, then prop your hands up on a chair or stable object and as you get stronger move your hands down to the floor: alternatively rest your knees on the floor (Fig 11). Once you can cope with these easily, start to elevate the legs finally reaching a position where you are doing them in a handstand position with your feet against a wall (Fig 12). Fingertip press-ups where you use your fingertips rather than the palms of your hands may be useful. One arm push-ups are a further way in which to increase the load, as is widening your hand and feet positions or keeping your elbows close to your sides.
2. *Dips* Start with your arms straight then lower your body until your elbow joint is at ninety degrees, then straighten your arms again. If you cannot do these with your legs in the air then let them touch the floor (Fig 13). Your legs should be controlled so that they do not assist with the action; quality is

better than quantity. Make sure that whatever you use to support yourself with is secure.
3. *Rope-wind* Hang a water bottle on a piece of string and attach this to a bar (an old broom handle 30cm long). Wind the weight (vary this by the amount of water in the bottle) up to the bar and unwind slowly. Repeat as necessary (Fig 14).
4. *Rope climb* In a gym you will frequently be able to find a rope suspended from the ceiling. Climb it, first using your feet and hands, then as you get fitter try without using your feet with your legs in the half-lever position (legs at ninety degrees to your trunk). To get the most out of this exercise climb down in control.
5. *Pull-ups (Fig 15)* You can usually find something to perform this exercise on though unless you are already quite strong you will find it hard to do very many, if any at all of these. As with the dips, resting your feet lightly on a support may help and as with the rope climb lower yourself slowly to receive maximum benefit from this exercise. Many gyms have a pull-up beam which has been adapted so that fingertip pull-ups can be achieved, alternatively door lintels can provide the same facility.
6. *Mantelshelves* Using a beam perform a series of mantelshelving movements. These can start from a hanging position or from the mid-point position so that you are only working upon the push part. If you try these on a beam you may experience some difficulty with your balance. It is easier to do them on to a box where your legs will be prevented from swinging below you. Do them with your fingers pointing forwards, towards each other and then turned outwards, as each of these will work the muscles differently.
7. *Laybacks* It is frequently possible to

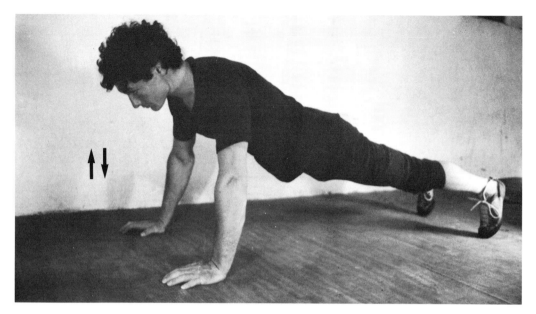

Fig 10 Press-ups.

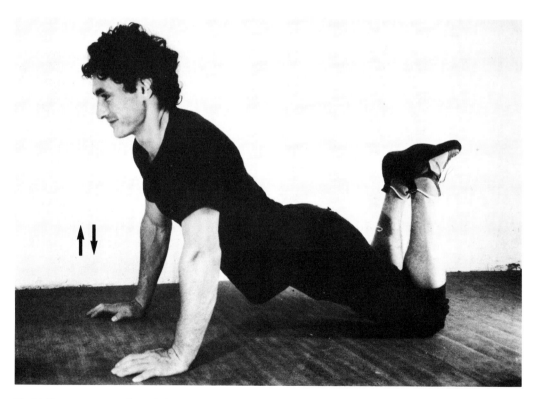

Fig 11 Press-ups; an easier variation.

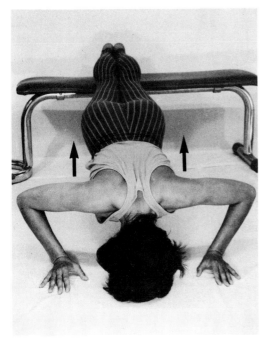

Fig 12 Press-ups; a harder variation.

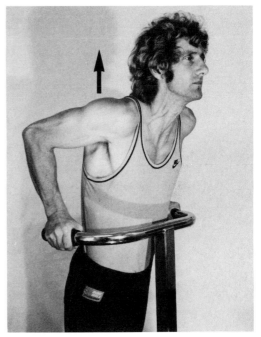

Fig 13 Dips.

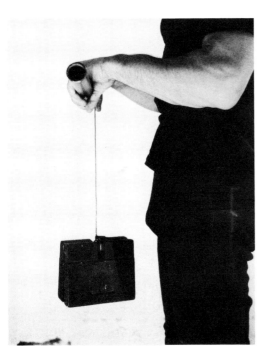

Fig 14 Rope wind (using weights).

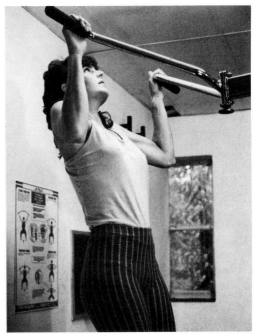

Fig 15 Pull-ups with palms forwards.

find apparatus in a gym on which you can perform laybacking manoeuvres, but be sure that you can do them sufficiently well to be able to maintain your pulse rate within the training zone.

8. *Ladders and wall bars* Climb these either using your feet or by letting them swing free.

9. *Lock-offs* Either using parallel ropes or slings suspended from a beam about a metre apart pull up, lock off and then repeatedly transfer from one to the other.

10. *Wrist flexing* With your arms extended, flex your wrist up and down, or in a circular fashion. If your heart rate drops out of the training zone during this exercise then do not include any more in this circuit.

11. *Shrugs* Using the same apparatus as with the dips, hold yourself up with your arms straight, including the wrist. Keeping your arms straight throughout, allow your body to sink down between your shoulders (it is important that you do this in control)

and then push up so that your head is as high as you can get it.

Middle Body

1. *Curls to the knees* Lying on your back, curl up so that your hands can reach the knees; do not go any further (Fig 16). As you lower yourself back to the floor do so in control unrolling your spine bit by bit on to the floor.

2. *Curls* Preferably with your feet held in position and your knees bent, curl up and touch your toes. As you get fitter perform the same manoeuvre with hands to the side of your head, but not behind as you can pull too hard on your neck. Adding a twist so that your left elbow touches your right knee and then your right elbow touches your left knee is also a good variation (Fig 17).

3. *Crunches* Elevate your legs so that when you lie on your back your knees are at ninety degrees. With your hands beside

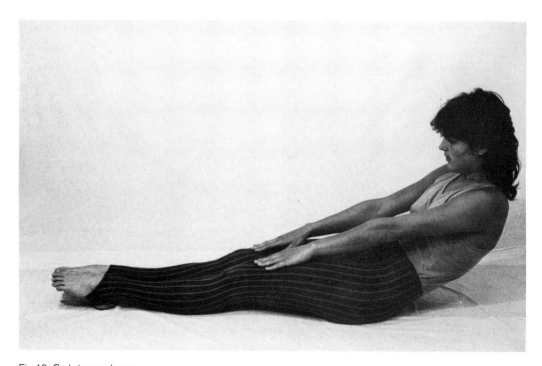

Fig 16 Curls to your knees.

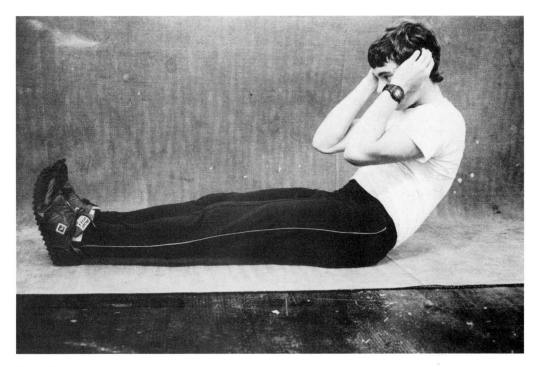

Fig 17 Curls.

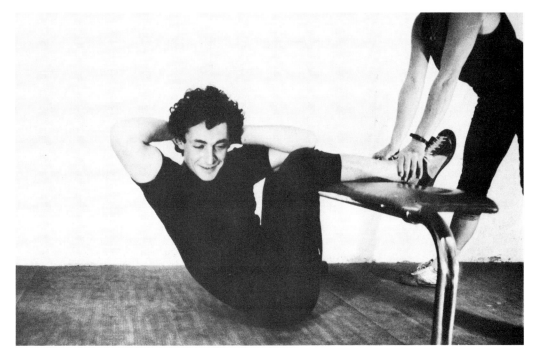

Fig 18 Crunches with a twist.

your head curl up. Again, the addition of a twisting element is good practice (Fig 18).

4. *Knee raises* With your body in the dips position or hanging from a bar, raise your knees towards your chest (Fig 19). As you get fitter try it with your legs out straight (Fig 20).

5. *Back extension* Lying on your stomach with your feet fixed and your hands behind your head, elevate your head by arching your back, as far as you can. These can also be done with the front half of your body hanging over the edge of a box (Fig 21).

6. *V-sits* Lying on your back lift both your legs and your trunk until you can touch your knees. Keep your legs and back straight throughout the manoeuvre (Fig 22).

Legs

1. *Shuttle runs* Runs back and forth between two markers.

2. *Squat jumps* Squat down, jump up.

3. *Squat thrusts* From the press-up position, keeping your hands on the floor, jump your feet up to your body (your knees should be outside your arms); jump them back to the original position immediately.

4. *Burpees* Same as above but stand up between squat thrusts.

5. *Step ups* Using a high bench step up and down with one leg leading. Repeat the same number on other leg.

6. *Straddle jumps* Standing astride a bench, jump up on to the bench and then back down again, and then repeat.

7. *Cross-over jumps* Starting on one side of the bench jump both legs over to the other side simultaneously.

8. *Knee raises* With your back to a wall raise each knee to your chest alternately.

9. *Tuck jumps* Jump up tucking your knees to your chest.

10. *Heel raises* With your toes raised about 10cm, keeping your legs straight, extend upwards (Fig 23). You can vary this by having your toes splayed outwards, parallel, or inwards (each exercise works on slightly different muscles). Once you can do

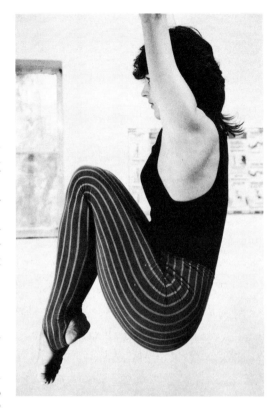

Fig 19 Knee raises.

these easily, try doing them with only one leg; doing them on a step with the heel hanging down low works the muscle over a larger range of movement and helps to stretch it.

WEIGHT TRAINING

Again we have divided the exercises into groups which apply to the major muscle groups being worked.

Upper Body and Shoulders

1. *Bench Press* This is great for upper body strength (Fig 24). A wide grip will emphasise the chest muscles and a narrow one the triceps and shoulder muscles.

Variations: (a) inclined press – this will alter the angle of muscle pull and will work

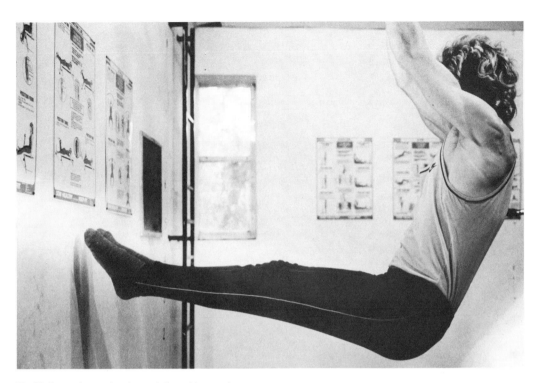

Fig 20 Leg raises; a harder variation of knee raises.

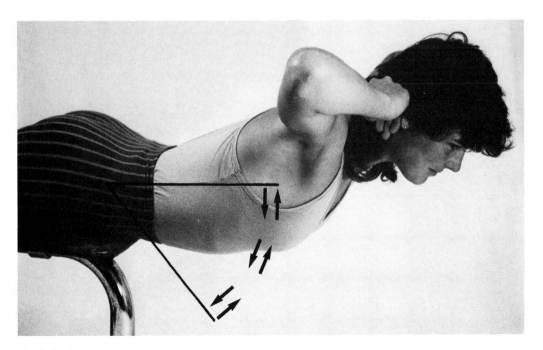

Fig 21 Back extension.

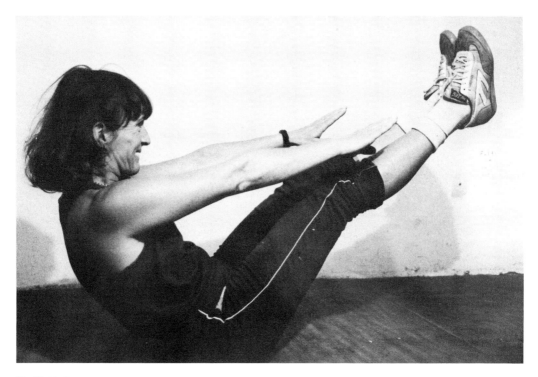

Fig 22 V-sits.

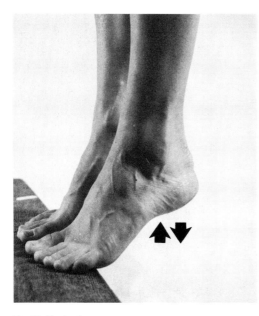

Fig 23 Heel raises.

the upper pectoralis muscles (Fig 25); (b) dumb-bells will involve more synergistic action and will also stretch the chest muscles more as the weight can be lowered below the chest line, each arm can be worked alternately or they can be worked at the same time (Fig 26).

2. *Shoulder press (Military press)* This, as its name suggests is excellent for the shoulders (Fig 27). Be very careful not to arch your back as this will strain the lower part of it.

Variations: (a) pressing behind the head will stress the muscles slightly differently and should be included occasionally to avoid staleness and for a more complete development; (b) again the dumb-bells can be raised alternately and the palms can be turned outwards or inwards to add variety. All the exercises can be done in a standing or seated position (Fig 28).

3. *Upright rows* Good for the trapezius, shoulders, arm flexors and upper chest. Keep the bar close to the body and do not

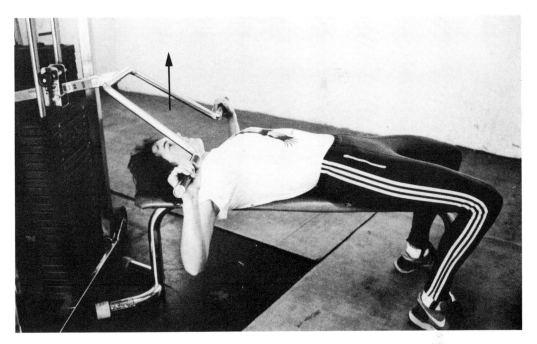

Fig 24 Bench press (do not hold your breath as your perform these).

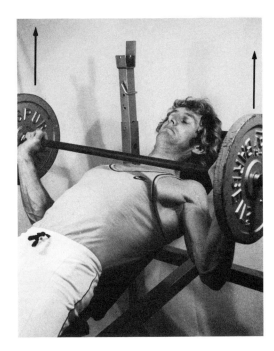

Fig 25 Inclined bench press.

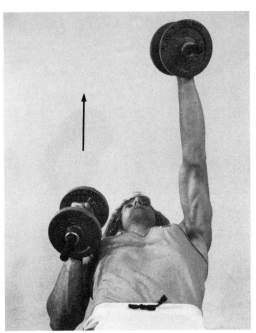

Fig 26 Bench press; with free weights.

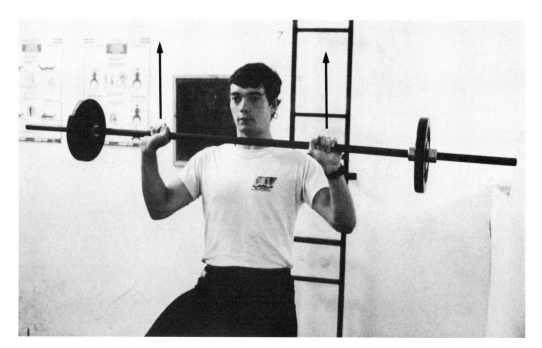

Fig 27 Shoulder press.

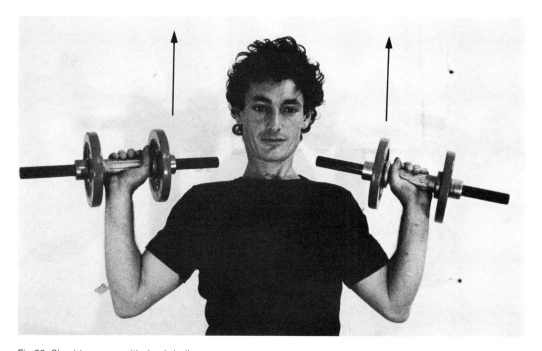

Fig 28 Shoulder press; with dumb-bells.

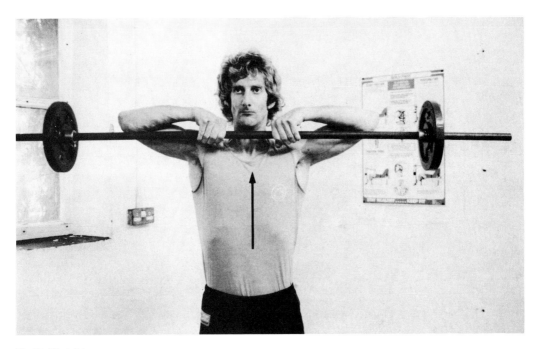

Fig 29 Upright rows.

bend your back. This exercise can be done with a variety of equipment (Fig 29).

4. *Lateral raises* These develop the outer head of the shoulders. Keep your arms slightly bent and use good form rather than trying to lift heavy weights (Fig 30).

5. *Front raises* These work the anterior deltoid muscles (Fig 31).

6. *Dips* These work many muscles – triceps, lats, anterior deltoids and pectorals. To be really effective, do them from a very low dipping position. With your elbows close to your sides you will work the triceps, and if you keep your chin on your chest and lean forwards throughout, at the same time as using a wider grip, you will work the chest muscles (*see* Fig 13).

7. *Lat pull-downs* Use a wide grip and keep your back slightly arched and your chest held high. Pull the elbows behind the body and never allow the chest to collapse. Pulling in front of the body is a rhomboideus and lattissimus movement and behind the body will involve the deltoids more (Fig 32).

8. *Chin ups* These are good for the upper back and the muscles involved in gripping.

Variations: by varying your grip both in the direction in which your palms face and in the width of your grip, you will work different parts of your lats. A wide grip works the upper lats and a narrow grip the lower lats (Fig 33).

9. *Dumb-bell bent rows* Good for the lattissimus muscles, and, because this exercise isolates the back, it can be used by those who have a back problem (Fig 34).

10. *Hyperextensions* These are good for the back extensors and do not place a stretching stress on the low back tendons and ligaments. It is not wise to go much beyond the parallel position as this could cause injury to the lower back (*see* Fig 21).

11. *Inverted flyes* The trapezius, rhomboideus, teres major, and infraspinatus all assist the posterior deltoids in this exercise (Fig 35).

12. *Pull-over* The elbows must be kept

47

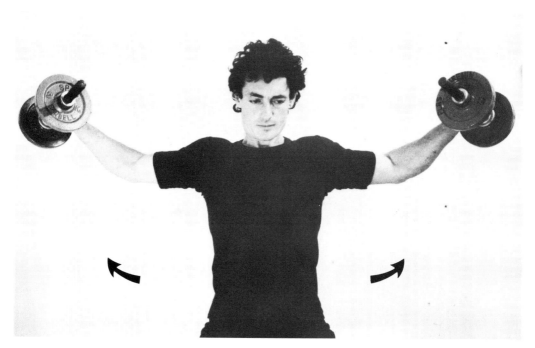

Fig 30 Lateral raises.

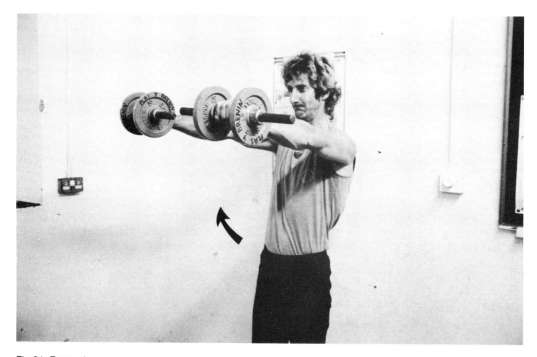

Fig 31 Front raises.

48

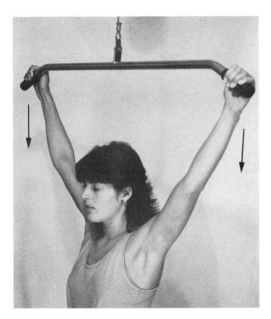

Fig 32 Lat pull-downs.

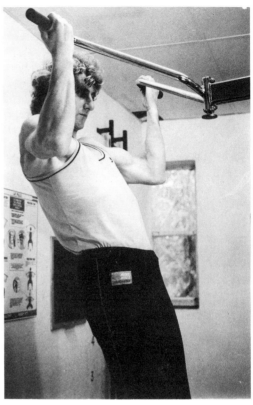

Fig 33 Chin-ups with a narrow grip (also known as pull-ups).

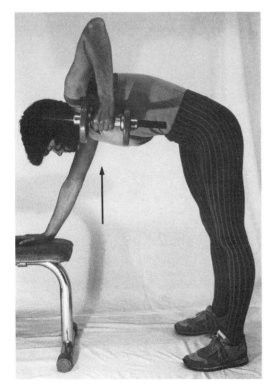

Fig 34 Dumb-bell bent rows.

pointing straight ahead and then the lats and triceps will be worked (Fig 36).

13. *Straight arm pull-over* Initially this works the lats but if you persist with it it will eventually strengthen the intercostals. The bar should be lowered far enough to stretch the lats and intercostals (Fig 37).

14. *Long pulley rows* These strengthen the middle trapezius and the rhomboideus as well as the elbow flexors (Fig 38).

15. *Triceps curls* There are many variations possible with this exercise, simply alter your grip and the position in which you do the exercise (Fig 39).

16. *Biceps curls* These can be done with a machine, bar or dumb-bells. The quality of movement is important. Be sure to keep your back straight throughout the movement (Figs 40 and 41).

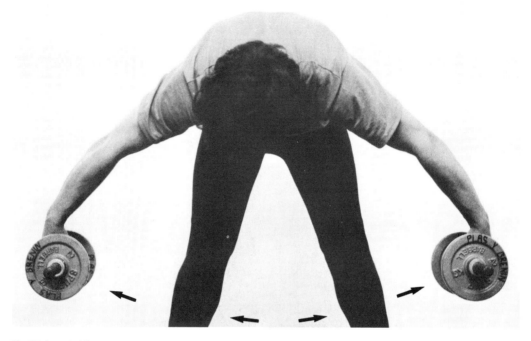

Fig 35 Inverted flyes.

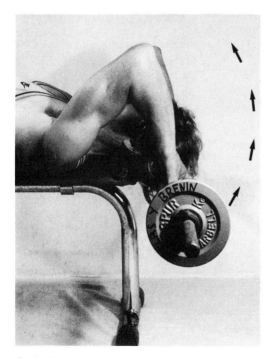

Fig 36 Pull-over.

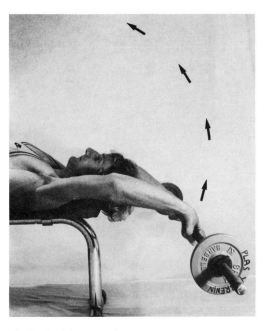

Fig 37 Straight arm pull-over.

Forearms and Hands

1. *Wrist curls* Support the forearm and curl wrist either with palms up or down; each works different muscles (Fig 42).
2. *Wrist rolling* Keep the arms out straight and work on the quality of the movement (Fig 43).
3. *Fingertip raises* Grip the rim of the plate with your fingers and raise and lower the plate (Fig 44).
4. *Plate grip* Using a smooth-sided plate, grip it between your thumb and fingers for 30 seconds (Fig 45).
5. *Squeezes* Most of the finger strength needed by climbers is in a static situation, so isometric exercises can be used, but remember that isometric work is very specific so be sure to work your fingers in a variety of positions. There are many things that can be used for squeezes; such as tennis balls, and it is rarely necessary to use specialised equipment.

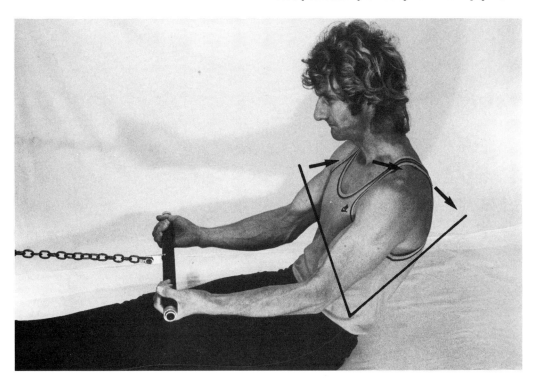

Fig 38 Long pulley rows.

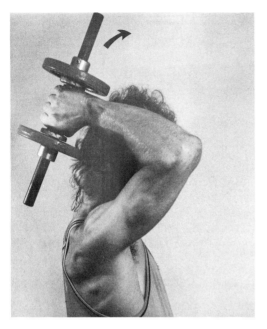

Fig 39 Triceps curls.

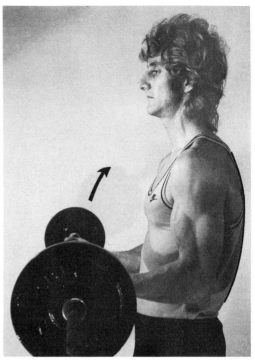

Fig 40 Biceps curls.

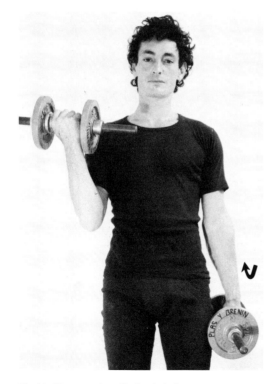

Fig 41 Biceps curls; with dumb-bells.

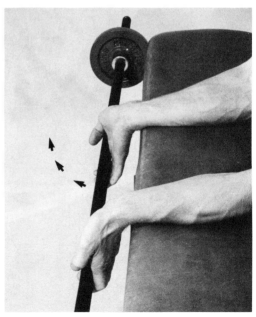

Fig 42 Wrist curls.

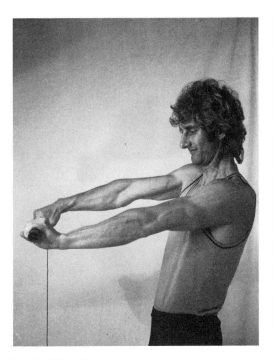

Fig 43 Wrist rolling.

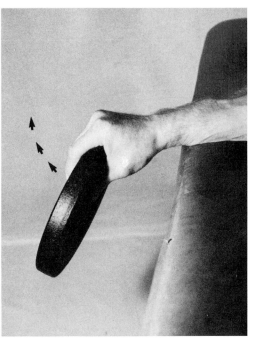

Fig 44 Fingertip raises.

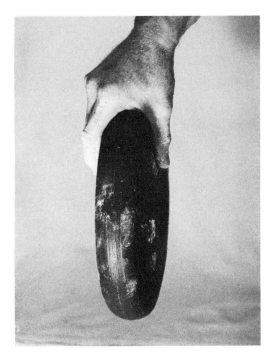

Fig 45 Plate grip.

Abdominals

These are the same as described without any apparatus but with the addition of an inclined sit-up board – the steeper the board the harder the work (Fig 46). In addition you can use the dip bar and raise the legs either in a bent position or with the legs straight.

Thighs

1. *Squats* In all squat movements be careful if you lower past the point at which your knee joint is at 90 degrees. If there is any sign of pain in or around the joint, stop.

Variations: you can have your feet flat, or heels raised and your feet in a wide stance (working inner thighs), or medium stance.

2. *Leg extensions* These are great for building the lower thigh and thus protecting the knee joint (Fig 47).

3. *Hamstring curls* Remember it is important to work these in order to get a balanced development of your legs (Fig 48).

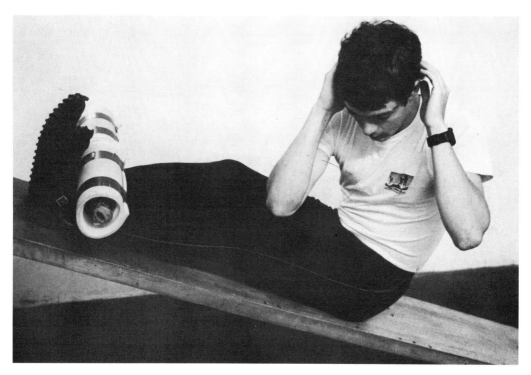

Fig 46 Inclined curls with a twist.

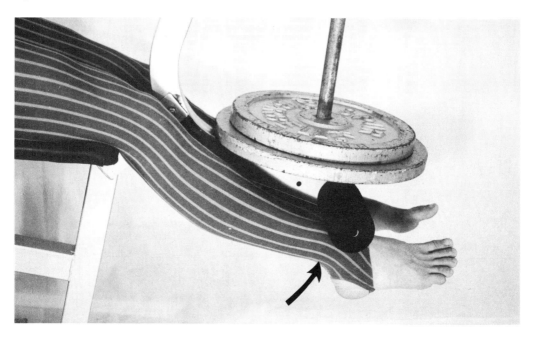

Fig 47 Leg extensions.

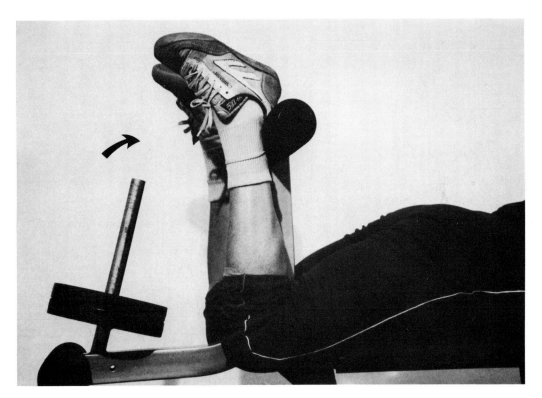

Fig 48 Hamstring curls.

4. *Leg press* This works the upper thighs – the same warning that was given with the squat applies here (Fig 49).

Hips

In all of these exercises it is vital to concentrate on a quality movement and at first signs of any pain in the knee joint you should stop. If your knees are susceptible to injury you can place the strap above the joint and continue in this fashion.

1. *Extensions* Keep your leg and back straight and extend your leg backwards (Fig 50).
2. *Flexions* Hold on to something in front of you and, keeping your leg straight, raise it as far as you can (Fig 51).
3. *Adductions* Supporting yourself at waist level bring your leg across in front of you (Fig 52a).

4. *Abductions* Keep the body upright and move the leg away from your body (Fig 52b).

Calves

1. *Heel raises* Using a board about two inches high the variations are numerous – both feet together, one at a time, with weights. By varying the angle of your feet (toes in, parallel, toes out) you will work slightly different parts of the muscle group. Some gyms have special machines designed for working the calves as it becomes difficult to load them sufficiently after a while. Donkey toe raises are another solution where you bend at the waist supporting yourself with your hands and get a partner to sit astride your hips.

This list of exercises is by no means totally comprehensive but you should find more than enough exercises to be able to work

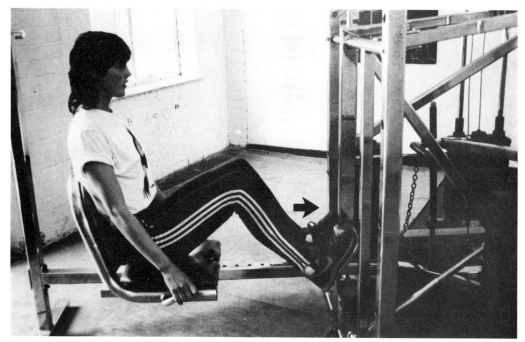

Fig 49 Leg press.

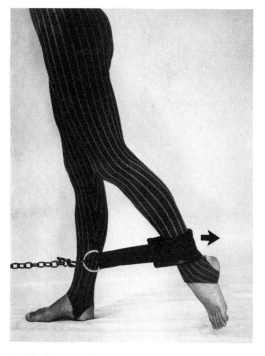

Fig 50 Hip extensions.

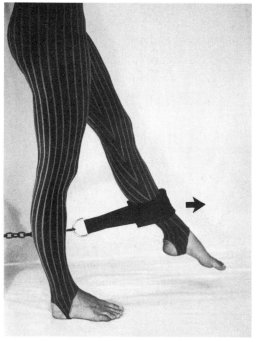

Fig 51 Hip flexions.

out a number of quite interesting programmes. For more ideas consult the references or your local gym.

FLEXIBILITY

These figures show the position you are aiming for. Do not cheat by twisting or curling as the stretch may then happen somewhere else. Follow the procedures, timings and repetitions outlined in chapter two.

1. *Side bends, spine and chest* (Fig 54). Keep the shoulders and hips facing forwards and the arms out at shoulder height. Slide the left hand down the left leg as you lift the right arm overhead, keeping it straight and close to your ear. Repeat other side.

2. *Shoulders* (Fig 55)

(a) Kneel or stand in front of a bench and fold from the hips so that your arms are straight, hands shoulder-width apart and palms down on the bench. Press down hard with your hands, count to 6 then relax, let your chest sink a little lower but keep your back straight.

(b) Grasp your hands, as shown, behind your head and hold for 30 seconds; repeat on both sides (Fig 56).

(c) Hold a broom handle with hands at a distance which allows you to move it overhead and behind, without twisting one shoulder through first. Bring it back to the front and repeat (Fig 57). You can easily monitor your improved shoulder flexibility by marking the stick where you hold it.

3. *Wrists and forearms* Kneel with hips above knees, shoulders above hands and turn your fingers towards your knees with

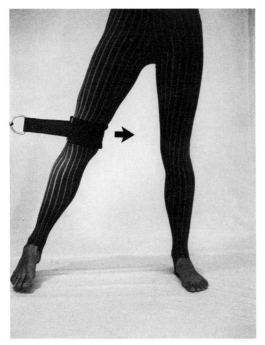

(a)

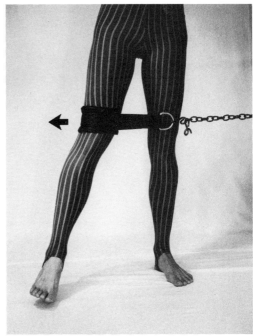

(b)

Fig 52 (a) Hip adductions; (b) hip abductions.

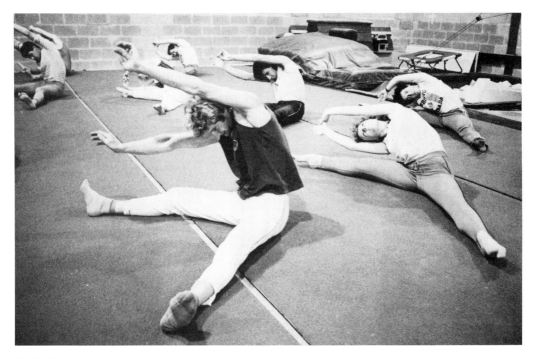

Fig 53 Stretching in a group can be fun. Notice the variations – stretch at your own level.

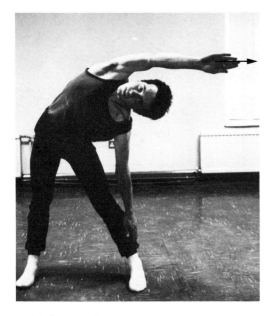

Fig 54 Side bends.

the palms facing down. Keeping your elbows straight lean back very carefully to stretch the forearm (Fig 58). Relax, circle the wrists and repeat. Turn your hands over so that the backs touch the floor, with the fingers pointing to your knees, straighten your elbows and hold. Relax and repeat (Fig 59).

4. *Quadriceps*

(a) Lie on your front with knees bent and grasp your ankles. Pull your feet towards you lifting the knees off the ground and hold (Fig 60). Rest and repeat.

(b) Kneeling on one knee, with your weight supported on your hands actively lift your other leg straight up behind you, do not jerk it. Lift and lower 10 times, then do the same with the other leg (Fig 61 – notice the variations in flexibility). This is also a strength exercise for the muscles doing the lifting.

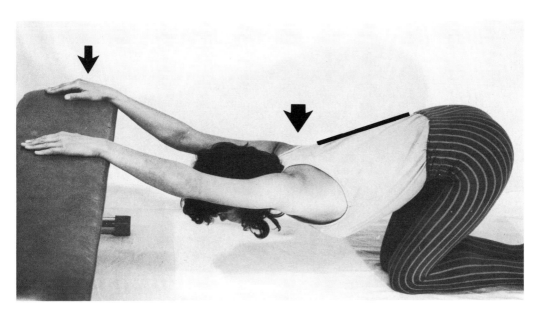

Fig 55 Shoulder stretch.

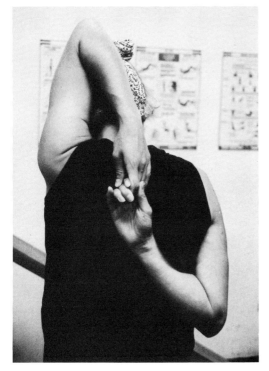

Fig 56 Triceps and shoulder stretch.

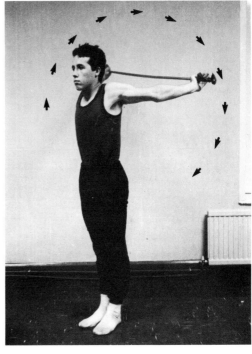

Fig 57 Broom handle stretch (you can also use a towel or better still a bicycle inner tube).

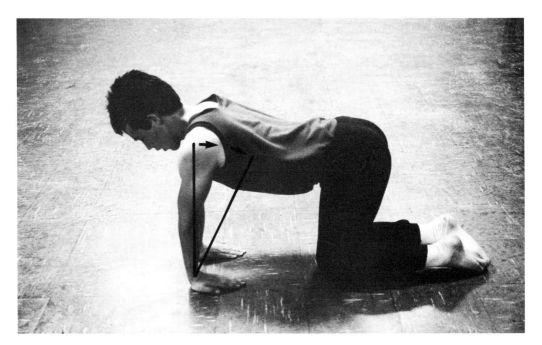

Fig 58 Forearm stretch.

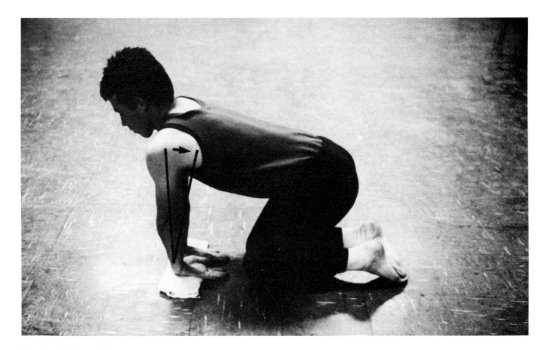

Fig 59 Wrist stretch.

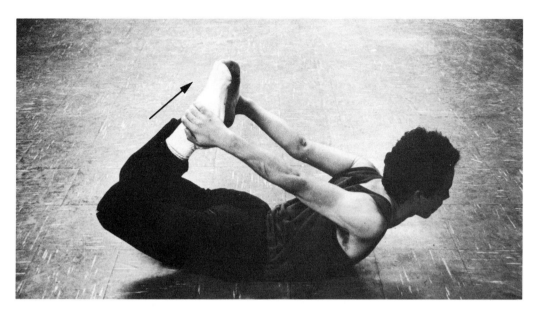

Fig 60 Quads stretch.

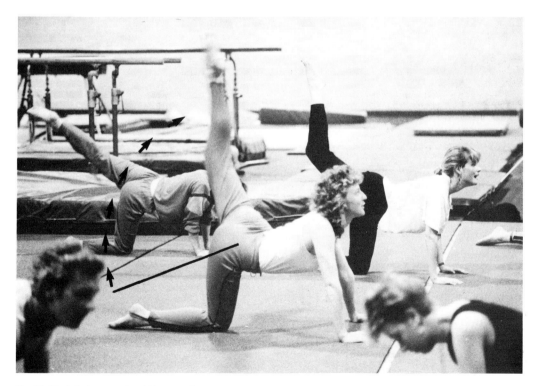

Fig 61 Straight leg quad and hip stretch.

5. *Abdomen*

(a) Lie prone, with hands beneath or a little in front of the shoulders, and keeping the thighs on the floor straighten your arms. Hold, roll down and repeat (Fig 62).

(b) Lie on your back with your feet on the floor close to you. Push your hips off the floor as high as possible, lower carefully and repeat.

6. *Shoulders, chest and buttocks* Hip roll – lie on your back with arms outstretched at shoulder level, palms down and knees tucked as tightly as possible to the chest. Keeping both shoulders on the floor, and the knees tucked up to the chest, roll your hips from left to right, aiming your knees in the direction of your armpit, 10 times each side (Fig 63 – this also strengthens your oblique abdominals).

7. *Hips and spine* Sit holding your ankles close to you, with the soles of your feet together, your pelvis tilted down at the front and your back straight or slightly arched. Rock on to the back of your pelvis as you curl forwards towards your feet, gently pushing down your knees with your elbows. Lift up your head first and uncurl your spine from top to bottom till you reach your starting position (Fig 64).

8. *Hips and hamstrings* (If you cannot sit with your back straight and your legs straight you will find this very awkward and not too beneficial, so it is best left till you have worked on hamstrings and hips individually – *see* exercises 7 and 10.)

(a) Sit in straddle position with a straight back and your arms up, in line with your body. Reach over to one side as far as you can with your top arm covering your ear, (do not fold forward), reach your hands towards your foot and come back up to the centre (Fig 65).

(b) Still in straddle position, sit, turn to face one leg and, keeping your arms in line

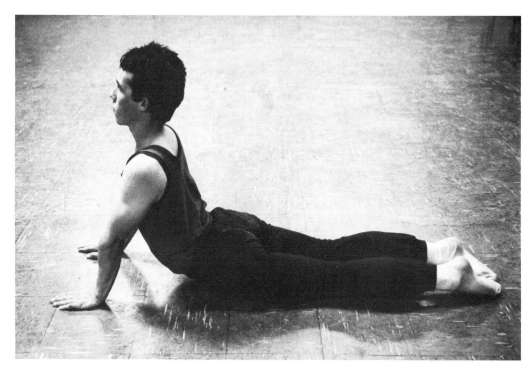

Fig 62 Abdomen stretch.

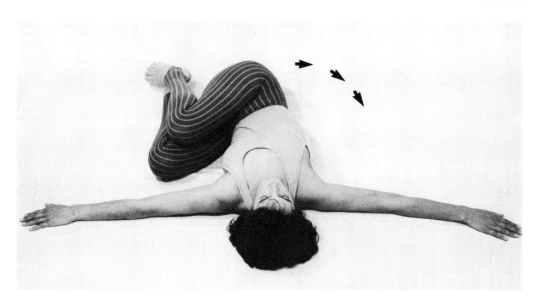

Fig 63 Hip roll.

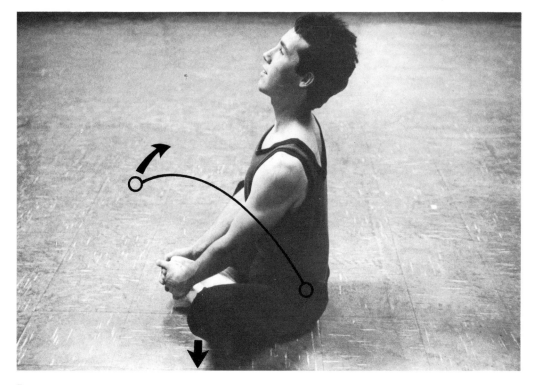

Fig 64 Hip stretch.

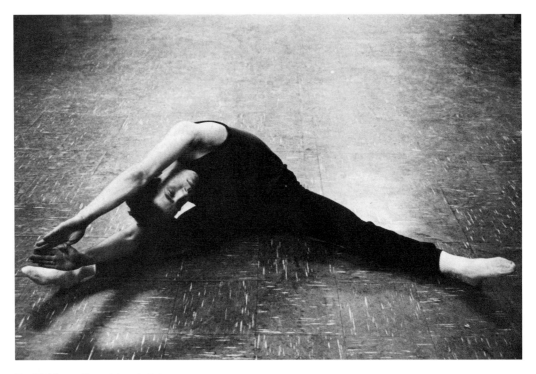

Fig 65 Hip and hamstring stretch.

with your body, lean forwards, aiming your lower ribs towards your thigh. If you press the back of your heel to the floor as you lower, you will control your weight and not stretch too rapidly. When you sit up, lift your arms first (Fig 66).

9. *Front of hips and hamstrings* Lunges – kneel up and place one foot forwards. With your hands behind your head and body upright, push your weight forwards so that you can lift your back knee off the floor. Keep that knee straight and push your heel backwards. You will feel the stretch behind the hip of the front leg and in the front of the other hip (Fig 67). Lower the back knee to the floor and straighten the front knee. Fold forward with a straight back and arms stretched behind, hold then pull the foot up towards your knee and hold again. 3 times each position, each leg. Do not be tempted to curl your spine, the object is not to get your head close to your leg but to achieve a tight fold at the hip (Fig 68).

10. *PNF on hamstrings* Lying on your back, your partner holds the leg at maximum stretch while you push against him for a count of 6. You both then relax and you move your leg to a closer angle at the hip before repeating twice (Fig 69). It is easier (for you and your helper) to do this in a sitting position if you are very stiff in the hamstrings. Make sure you sit with your back straight and do not allow your hips to slide out from the wall (Fig 70).

11. *Splits (with aid)* With hips square, both legs straight and the toes of your back leg turned under, place your hands on a bench or box between your legs and carefully lower your hips as you slide your feet apart. Both legs must stay straight. When you reach a position of maximum stretch, hold it and then repeat on alternate leg (Fig 71).

12. *Inner thigh*

(a) With a bench for stiff people, or with

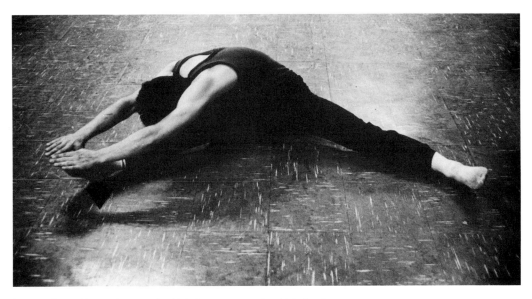

Fig 66 Hip and hamstring stretch with twist, press your heel into the floor.

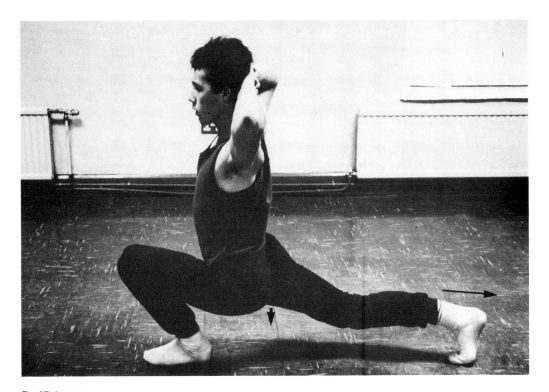

Fig 67 Lunges.

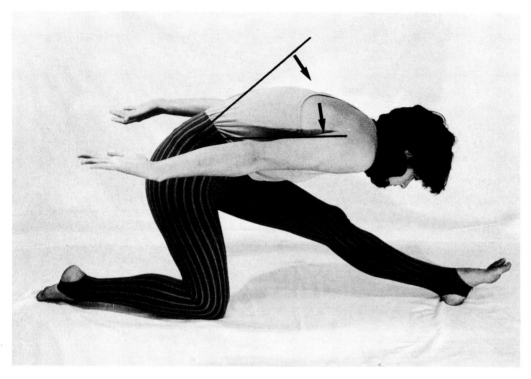

Fig 68 Hamstring stretch.

your hands on the floor, slide your feet out to the sides, keeping knees straight, and toes and knees turned up to the ceiling (if you do not rotate the legs out, there will be too much strain on the inner side of the knee joint). Press the heels against the floor, count to 6 then relax and slide your feet out a little; repeat twice more (Fig 72). If you have a helper, this PNF can be performed with you on your back. The helper holds the legs apart at the knee (not below it) and you try hard to close the legs together while your helper keeps them still. You both count to 6, then relax and you move both legs out to a wider position. Repeat from this new position and again from the next position (Fig 73).

(b) From a kneeling position with one leg out to the side of your knee and the leg straight, hands supporting in front, lift the leg high to the side and lower, 10 each side (Fig 74).

13. *Lower leg (back)* From a hands and knees position on the floor, straighten your legs and lift to a 'tent' position. Keeping knees straight, push your weight back and your heels towards the floor (note how far back the shoulders move), hold and then return to knees and rest, then repeat (Fig 75). For stiff people, sit with a scarf to reach round your feet and gently pull them up towards you, press against the scarf with the ball of the foot but do not let it move. Hold for 6, relax and repeat (Fig 76).

14. *Lower leg (side)* Stand with feet apart and parallel or turned in. Fold forwards and reach both hands as far to the side as possible (Fig 77).

15. *Rock and roll* At the end of a session relax and unwind. From a sitting position hugging your knees, roll back and forwards three times, then release your hands, reach them forwards and stand up (Fig 78).

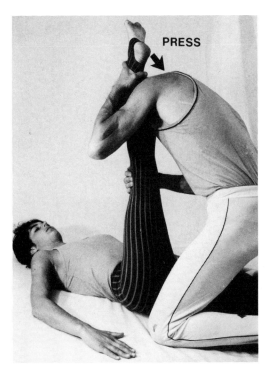

Fig 69 PNF hamstring stretch.

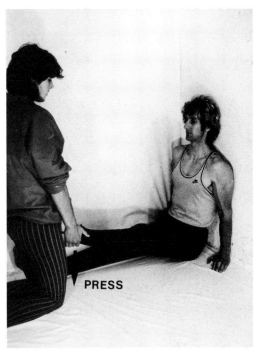

Fig 70 PNF hamstring stretch, a variation for less supple people.

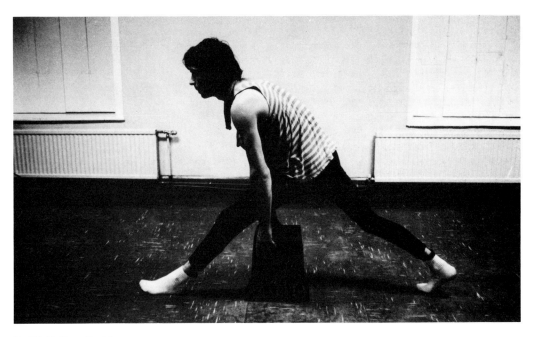

Fig 71 Splits, with aid.

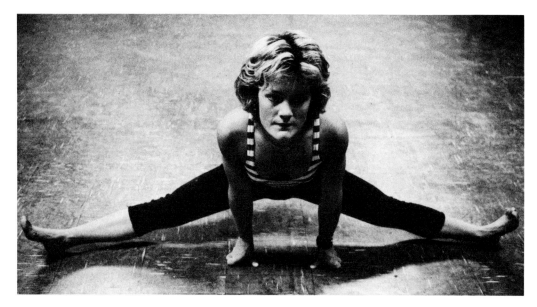

Fig 72 Inner thigh stretch.

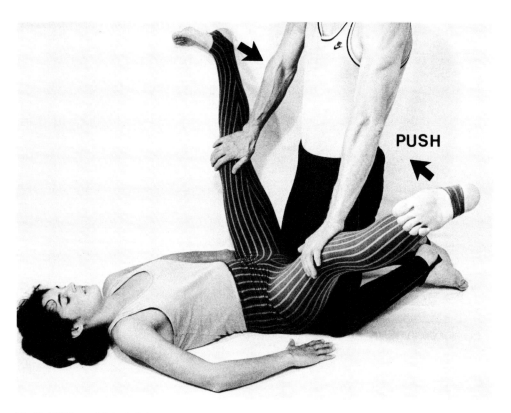

PUSH

Fig 73 PNF inner thigh stretch.

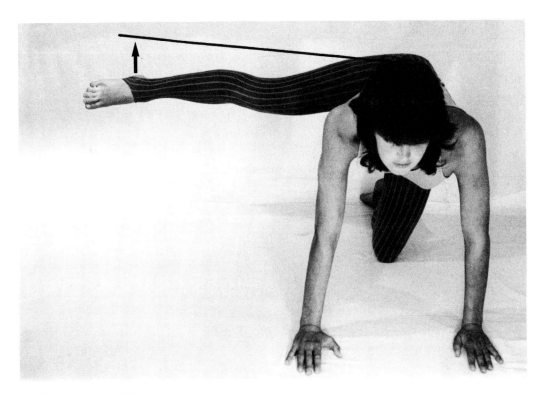

Fig 74 Inner thigh stretch.

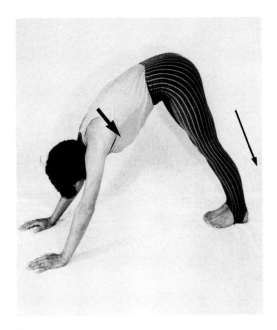

Fig 75 Lower leg, tent stretch.

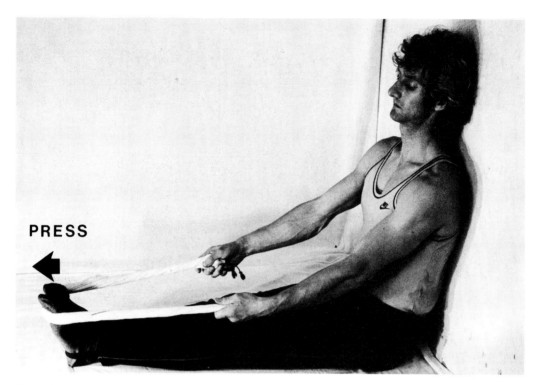

PRESS

Fig 76 Scarf stretch.

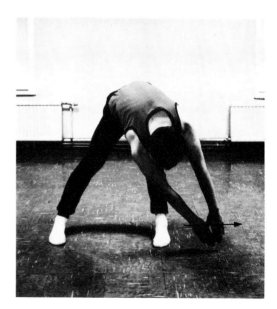

Fig 77 Lower leg side stretch.

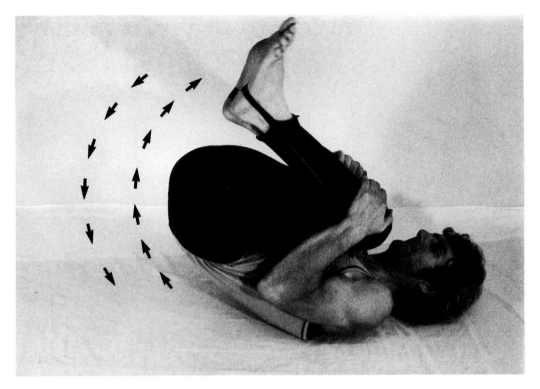

Fig 78 Rock and roll.

4 Programmes

One of the most important factors to consider in designing an appropriate fitness programme is deciding your exact needs, what you actually want to gain out of all this hard work. An awareness of some of the different areas of fitness and of their relevance to climbing will help you to make this decision.

ENDURANCE

Endurance can be divided into overall endurance and local muscular endurance; both utilise the following systems.

1. Aerobic fitness An increase in this system will raise the anaerobic threshold (the point at which the anaerobic system is employed). Work on this system will improve your overall fitness and health. It is the primary system for the Alpinist to develop, and although the rock climber relies heavily upon the anaerobic systems it is very important that time is spent on raising the anaerobic threshold, particularly as you embark upon a programme.
2. Anaerobic fitness
   (a) Phosphagen or alactic system. Training can improve this system by up to 300 per cent, and it can provide penalty-free energy (no fatigue) for up to 20 seconds of low grade anaerobic work. This may well be sufficient time to pass short intense cruxes on a rock climb, though whether it is this system that would be employed would depend upon the previous work-load. Obviously it is very difficult to generalise about the length of crux sections, but if you are climbing at a standard where you are getting pumped over short sections then this type of training would be worth trying alongside the others.

   (b) Glycolysis or lactic system. This system can provide energy for a period of between 50 seconds to 2 minutes (depending upon the work-load), but the penalties are high because the lactic acid that is produced by this system causes fatigue. This is the system employed during a rock climb where being pumped is a frequent occurrence. When training this system, try to work out whether you naturally have a predominance of fast twitch muscle fibres or slow twitch muscle fibres and train appropriately.

STRENGTH

Strength is the ability of a muscle to produce force. There is a tendency to exaggerate the need for strength, and perhaps some confusion arises over the difference between being unable to make a particular move because you are fatigued and need to train your local muscular endurance, and having insufficient strength. It is more likely to be the former. Strength training should be highly specific, but do remember to work the antagonistic muscles as well as this will help to avoid injuries and create a more balanced performance.

Power is the ability of a muscle to produce a force explosively and speedily. Increasingly, at the top end of the sport, this is becoming important. If you are able to climb quickly, you will spend less time in a position that tires you and will therefore use less lactic energy and not fatigue as quickly. Also, we are seeing more and more use of dynamic climbing techniques which are very explosive and it may be that plyometric training principles will be of value here.

FLEXIBILITY

This area of fitness concerns the mobility of our bodies – the importance of this to the climber is apparent to most. A flexible body not only allows you to reach holds but allows you to use them more efficiently, thereby taxing the muscles less. In addition, stretching should form an integral part not only of your training programme but also your day's climbing, as this will help to prevent injuries. A wise climber will warm up properly before embarking on the route and part of this warm-up should include some stretching.

EXAMPLE PROGRAMMES

The following are example programmes for a variety of different people. It is vital that, with the knowledge you have gained from the previous chapters, you analyse your own requirements as honestly as possible, throwing out any preconceived ideas, and adapt these very basic programmes to suit your individual needs. These needs will be governed by your aspirations as a climber and the availability of both a training place and training time. It must also be remembered that climbing at the limit of your ability is the best training of all except in a very few exceptional cases.

The concept behind these programmes is known as periodisation and whilst we accept that most of you will be climbing the year round we also recognise that there are seasons within climbing, periods when you will want to see your performance peak, and this form of programming will help you to do that. If you want to peak twice (winter ice and summer rock for example) then condense the layout of these programmes into six-monthly periods or whatever is appropriate.

Period one is usually the warm-up period, especially applicable to those new to training. Period two is the off-season phase, lasting 6 to 8 weeks. It is the time to maintain or start to build your aerobic fitness. Some strength training is appropriate here because it reduces the chore of very intensive pre-season training. If you have recognised weaknesses in your performance, then this is the time to start to build them up – though not at the expense of your strengths. There are some people who believe that you should not concentrate on your weaknesses at all but rather build upon your strengths. We, however, recommend the more balanced approach outlined first.

Period three is the pre-season phase (6–8 weeks) where, if the previous training has been correct, you can bring yourself to peak fitness. The intensity of the exercises will be increased and it will be necessary to specify very closely. Anaerobic work can also reach full intensity, although it must be noted that there are real problems of physiological and psychological fatigue if anaerobic training is carried out for too long – this will also increase the likelihood of injury.

Period four is the in-season phase where most of the training is of a maintenance variety – fortunately, although all forms of fitness are reversible, one can maintain levels of fitness with a lower level of intensity than was necessary to reach that stage. Generally the longer the build-up to a level of fitness, the longer it takes to lose it.

The final period is the post-activity phase or warm-down. It is a period of active rest with some low intensity, mainly aerobic, work. It should rest you both physiologically and psychologically. You should think of the rest periods as being as important as any of the others, because it is during these periods that your body undergoes the physiological changes that are the result of all your efforts. If you do not rest properly then your body has insufficient time to recuperate and you will actually lose fitness, and may even suffer injury (*see* Fig 79).

Each programme includes an annual breakdown and a weekly programme for each phase. The weekly programmes indicate the intensity you should be aiming for during each session and some of them,

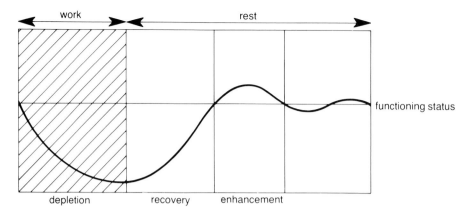

The pattern of work

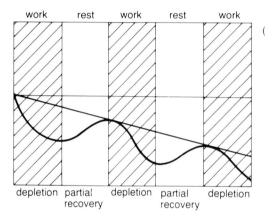

(a) If you do not rest sufficently, your level of fitness will not increase.

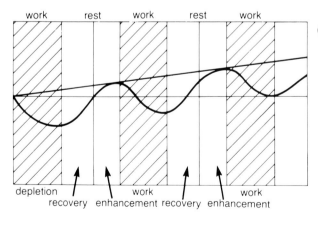

(b) Correct rest periods will lead to an increase in fitness.

Fig 79 The pattern of work, debilitation and enhancement, showing the importance of correctly spaced rest periods (all three graphs are different scales). Unless you allow your body to rest, your level of fitness may deteriorate, and if you rest too much your fitness will not improve.

particularly at the higher levels, include rotas for ten-day periods or longer. They assume that most of you will be climbing at the weekends – if this is not the case then adapt them appropriately. To determine the actual amounts of work and specific exercises, refer to the previous relevant chapters.

Finally, remember to keep some sort of record of your progress as this is the key to making all the hard work effective. If you do not achieve the results you want, you will need to change your programme and you can only do this effectively if you have kept a detailed account of what you have been doing.

Programme 1: Alpinism (medium intensity)

Jan	Feb	Mar	Apr	May	Jun	Jul	Aug	Sep	Oct	Nov	Dec
[One]											
	[········Two·········]										
			[······· Three ········]								
					[····Activity····]						
							[········Rest·······]				

Period One

This period will be spent on building up your general aerobic fitness. Start with some simple runs lasting about 20–30 minutes, 3 times a week. Record your resting pulse rate and see how it drops. Gradually increase the distance so that you are keeping your heart rate in the training zone for 30 minutes. Stretch before and after exercise.

Weekly Programme

Intensity	medium		hard		medium	light	light
	Monday	**Tuesday**	**Wednesday**	**Thursday**	**Friday**	**Saturday**	**Sunday**
Activity	stretch run stretch	rest	stretch run stretch	rest	stretch run stretch	normal climbing & walking weekend	

Period Two

In this period add some variety to your programme by introducing some fartlek sessions, and maybe towards the end some circuit training. Both of these elements will continue to increase your general level of aerobic fitness, but will also allow you to specify more closely. Your legs will need to be doing most of the work, but do not neglect the other parts of your body. Again, do no more than three sessions a week and be careful to consider your weekends and the effect they have; if they are active then they can form one of the sessions. You may decide to add some local muscular work now in the form of calf work for cramponing and thigh exercises to strengthen the muscles around the knee, which will help to prevent injuries of that joint. Cycling in a high gear, provided you back it up with some work on your hamstrings, could also be useful to build the thigh muscles. This type of work should only be introduced towards the middle of this period.

Weekly Programme

Intensity	medium/hard		hard		medium	medium	light
	Monday	**Tuesday**	**Wednesday**	**Thursday**	**Friday**	**Saturday**	**Sunday**
Activity	stretch fartlek stretch	rest	stretch circuits stretch	rest	stretch cycle stretch	climbing and walking	active rest

Add the calf and thigh work as necessary.

Period Three

It is now time to lengthen the training sessions. Start by including at least one long slow run (1 hour building up to 2 hours), and add others providing you are recovering properly. Long walks or climbs with sacks should form a major part of the final stages of this programme. Any anaerobic and strengthening exercises should be reaching their full intensity at this stage.

Weekly Programme

Intensity		medium		hard		hard	medium
	Monday	**Tuesday**	**Wednesday**	**Thursday**	**Friday**	**Saturday**	**Sunday**
Activity	rest	stretch long slow run stretch	rest	stretch circuits stretch	rest	long walks and climbs with sacks stretch	

Programme 2: Alpinism (high intensity)

Only embark on this programme if you are already fit.

Jan	Feb	Mar	Apr	May	Jun	Jul	Aug	Sep	Oct	Nov	Dec
								[· · ·One · · ·]			
									[· · · · · · · · · · · ·Two· ·		
· · · · · · ·]											
	[· · · · · · · · · · · · · ·Three · · · · · · · · · · · · · ·]										
					[· · · · · · · · ·Activity· · · · · · · · ·]						

Period One

This is only necessary if you have not been training for a while. If this is the case, proceed as in the previous example. If, however, you have just finished an Alpine season then we would suggest that you take a rest during this period, hence the overlap with the activity phase in the above chart.

Period Two

This is a longer and more intense repetition of the same ideas expressed in the previous example.

Weekly Programme

Intensity	hard		hard		hard	medium	light
	Monday	**Tuesday**	**Wednesday**	**Thursday**	**Friday**	**Saturday**	**Sunday**
Activity	stretch fartlek stretch	rest	stretch circuits stretch	rest	stretch cycle stretch	climbing and walking	active rest

Add the calf and thigh work as necessary.

Period Three

Again a repeat of the previous example but with greater intensity.

Weekly Programme

Intensity		hard		hard		hard	hard
	Monday	**Tuesday**	**Wednesday**	**Thursday**	**Friday**	**Saturday**	**Sunday**
Activity	rest	stretch long slow run stretch	rest	stretch circuits stretch	rest	long walks and climbs with sacks	

Programme 3: Rock Climbing (relative newcomers)

Jan	Feb	Mar	Apr	May	Jun	Jul	Aug	Sep	Oct	Nov	Dec
Climb					Climb					Climb	

We do not mean this glibly – at this stage of your climbing the best training has to be climbing. If you must train then follow a general programme of fitness training.

Programme 4: Rock Climbing (medium intensity)

Jan	Feb	Mar	Apr	May	Jun	Jul	Aug	Sep	Oct	Nov	Dec
									[···One···]		
											[·····Two··
·······]											
	[·····Three·····]										
		[························· Four ······················]									

Period One

In the warm-up period for this programme, the work is entirely aerobic, and the best medium is usually running. The object is to improve the cardio-respiratory system.

Depending upon how fit you are to start with, this period can last from 2 weeks (for those who are already fit) to 6 weeks (for those who are just starting a programme). If you are into your second year then this period should be one of active rest.

Weekly Programme

Intensity	medium		hard		medium	light	light
	Monday	**Tuesday**	**Wednesday**	**Thursday**	**Friday**	**Saturday**	**Sunday**
Activity	stretch run stretch	rest	stretch run stretch	rest	stretch run stretch	normal climbing weekend	

Period Two

Having improved your cardio-respiratory system and raised your anaerobic threshold in the process, you should now start to specify and work on some local muscular endurance – though during this period we suggest that you continue to work the whole body. Circuit training and the use of weights can be introduced at this point. If you are able to use a wall (or boulders) then use it for skills training before your training session, but after the stretching on Monday and Wednesday.

Weekly Programme

Intensity	hard		medium		medium	hard	light
	Monday	**Tuesday**	**Wednesday**	**Thursday**	**Friday**	**Saturday**	**Sunday**
Activity	stretch fartlek run stretch	stretch	stretch circuits or weights stretch	stretch	stretch circuits stretch	climb	climb

Introduce some specific strength training if necessary.

Period Three

In this period we suggest that you maintain your aerobic fitness and start to specify on the upper body. Apart from some strength training where required, the work should at this level remain aerobic, with an increase in the skills learning use of the wall or bouldering. If it is possible then use your wall for some aerobic training as well.

Weekly Programme

Intensity		hard		hard		hard	medium
	Monday	**Tuesday**	**Wednesday**	**Thursday**	**Friday**	**Saturday**	**Sunday**
Activity	stretch	stretch wall (skills) circuits stretch	stretch	stretch wall (aerobic) weights stretch	stretch	climb	climb

Period Four

You will basically be climbing during this period but remember to maintain your level of fitness.

Programme 5: Rock Climbing (high intensity)

Jan	Feb	Mar	Apr	May	Jun	Jul	Aug	Sep	Oct	Nov	Dec
									[···One···]		
										[·····Two··
······]											
	[····Three····]										
		[······················Four··············]									

This programme assumes a very high level of residual fitness and commitment to the sport and it therefore can only be a rough guide since we asssume that you will climb at every opportunity.

Period One

Rest. There must be a period of rest – it can be active rest, for example, easier climbs, but it must be stressed that at this level of commitment the biggest risk is that you will over-train. Remember it is during the rest periods that your body adapts, and they are therefore the most important periods in the whole schedule. Without them your body will not change, your level of fitness will not improve and injuries will result.

Period Two

Having analysed your performance carefully and honestly you should be able to decide which areas you want to work upon. In this period you should work on improving your aerobic fitness both generally and specifically, hence the need for runs and circuits. It is also a good time to work on strength if you feel it is appropriate, although the chances are that it is not likely at this stage in your climbing. Physiologically, work on the wall (or boulders) should be mainly aerobic, though psychologically you may want to use the wall for skills training not to mention just plain fun!

Weekly Programme

Intensity	hard		medium		medium	hard	light
	Monday	**Tuesday**	**Wednesday**	**Thursday**	**Friday**	**Saturday**	**Sunday**
Activity	stretch fartlek run stretch	stretch	stretch circuits or weights stretch	stretch	stretch circuits stretch	climb	climb

Introduce some specific strength training if necessary.

You will notice that at this stage the programme is the same as the one used in programme 4, the only difference being that you will probably be working with harder exercises.

Period Three

To get the most out of this period you will have to analyse your needs very carefully because this will be the time to introduce such concepts as plyometrics and anaerobic training. It is going to be a period of high specialisation and as such demands great care on your part if you are to prevent injuries. Listen to your body very carefully, and at the first signs of any undue discomfort, particularly in the joints, rest that particular area. If you do decide to include any anaerobic training in this period then try to decide which is the most appropriate form – careful record-keeping will again aid you in getting the best results from your work. Because of the specialisation that is required at this level of performance, we feel that it is pointless to suggest a typical weekly programme and in fact a longer cycle may be more useful. To give you an idea of these we have included one, but it must be stressed that you should by now be able to design your own and it would be better to do so.

DAY	1	2	3	4	5	6	7	8	9	10
I	H	H	R	R	M	R	H	H	R	R
	S	S	S	S	S	S	S	S	S	S
	R				F		R			
		W	W(s)			W(s)		W		
	AN				AN		AN			
		C						C		
	S	S	S		S	S	S	S		

Key: I – Intensity, H – Hard, M – Medium, R – Rest
S – Stretching
R – Run
F – Fartlek run

W – Wall
W(s) – Wall (skills training only)
AN – Anaerobic work
C – Circuits

5 Mental Training

In many sports, the athlete's mind is now considered to be the 'last performance frontier'. Most climbers, at whatever level, have realised that their mind plays an incredibly important role in the outcome of a climb. We have long recognised that the top climbers of the day are not necessarily the fittest and that it is their control and mental attitude that allow them to succeed where other fitter and stronger climbers have failed. Although the attitudes of these climbers are as varied as the climbs themselves, there are a number of common factors that prevent us from performing to the best of our ability whatever the sport. The techniques that enable us to make the most of our level of skill and suppress the factors that inhibit performance are discussed in detail in this chapter.

Many climbers may be worried at the thought of tampering with their thought processes but, as Hardy points out, in *How can we help performers?*:

'the self regulation skills which mental training provides will not mean that you become some sort of robot who no longer experiences such emotions as fear or joy at success. Rather they will enable you to contain the effects of these emotions so that they do not affect your immediate performance or threaten your immediate well being.'

It is also essential to understand that the ideas expressed in this chapter are no short cut to the top echelons of the sport but require as much perseverance and training as the physical programmes outlined earlier. Thought processes are as varied as the bodies they control so not all of these ideas will be applicable to you. Some will be, so choose these and work on them with the same dedication that you apply to your physical workouts. Many of them can be integrated into your normal routines but, like physical training, they have to be specific to your needs and situation.

GOAL SETTING

The goal which you set for yourself must be realistic and should be divided into three different types. (These are the categories described by W. Railo.)

1. The Training Controller This is a realistically evaluated objective based on an honest appraisal of your total ability and level of ambition. It will be the one which dictates your training programme and presupposes a development towards harder climbs. But this alone is not enough because there is a risk of mental blocks and of performance anxiety (caused by not meeting your goals), therefore the following types are also used.
2. The Barrier Breaker The danger in setting a goal is that once you have reached it you will find it hard to pass. By mental training, you can condition your subconscious to accept better results and thereby prevent a barrier from being formed.
3. The Security Builder This is vitally important because failure to achieve your goal can have a very negative effect. It is necessary to anticipate this and prepare yourself for it through mental training.

Numbers two and three can be accomplished through the use of visualisation techniques. Goal setting can be long term ('I am a severe climber and I want to be climbing HVS by the end of the summer') or short term ('I want to get to the top of this pitch'). In both cases the end goal can be very daunting, so it is useful to divide it up into shorter approachable units. Many experienced climbers are well practised at this skill but if you are relatively new to the sport then it is something you will have to work on. Concentrate on the first ten feet and get up that, then concentrate on the next ten feet and so on. Gradually you will be able to cope with bigger and bigger distances without them creating negative feelings. Changing negative responses into positive ones and always trying to be positive is what confidence building is all about.

CONFIDENCE BUILDING

Systematic conscious positive thinking will make your reactions positive, and it is necessary to work on this in all of your training. Negative reactions can also be learned, and these reactions have become known as the 'fight or flight' response. The fight response is positive, but it is very important to remember that it is *not* aggressive, and the flight response is negative. To fight is to maintain your self-confidence and to keep to your objectives; the flight reaction on the other hand is to try to escape mentally from the situation ('I am not good at jamming cracks', 'I have not been training much recently', 'I do not like limestone' and so on). We all recognise this type of behaviour to some degree or another, but to change it we must change our attitude and be more on the offensive ('I *can* climb jam cracks'). This is quite different from being aggressive. Aggression is directed by the emotions, whereas the person who is on the offensive is merely committed to the task in hand in a confident and positive way. Obviously you must be motivated for the task and this is where it is important to strengthen your will-power. It is will-power that enables you to climb jamming cracks or limestone even if you do not like them. In sports like climbing where endurance is very important, will-power is very signi-

ficant and you can start to train it during your physical training sessions. Start in a small way by not giving up in exercises until you have achieved your goals (except where to continue would mean injury). Make these goals reasonable and not too ambitious at the beginning, then build on your success. Training the will-power is a long term project.

RELAXATION

First we must answer the question 'Why do we need special methods in order to relax?' After all, many people have turned to climbing because the intensity of the activity is so absorbing that it acts as a means of relaxing, a means of escaping from the everyday pressure of life. However, the ability to stop yourself from 'tightening up', is crucial not only when you are climbing, but also when you are training and especially in order to get the most out of your mental training. A relaxed mind is more receptive to the processes of mental training. To attain a peak performance you must be correctly aroused – too little or too much will result in you not performing to your full potential. The ability to relax means that you can control the level of arousal, especially if it gets too high (a frequent occurence for many of us when we are climbing). You will probably appreciate this if you recall the feeling you get just after placing protection in a steep and exposed position. Before placing it you feel fatigued, your arms are aching, and your breathing is heavy, but as soon as the protection has been placed you are able to relax, your arms ache less and your breathing becomes controllable; the tension of the situation causes most of the problems.

There are many different methods and techniques available and different ones will suit different people because of the ways in which our brains tend to function. This is a complex area that is constantly being revised in the light of new research findings, but basically the two hemispheres of our brains appear to control different types of behaviour. The left is analytical, logical and verbal whereas the right is artistic, intuitive and spatial. Most people are reasonably able to switch from one to the other but many will have a preferred mode and this is why you will find some relaxation techniques easier to use than others. A few that you may find useful are outlined here.

Breathing

You may be aware that when you are under stress you tend to use the upper part of your chest and its associated muscles to breath with, whereas when you are relaxed most of the action seems to take place down towards the abdomen. By controlling your breathing and trying to use your stomach muscles you may find yourself more relaxed. This is a very useful technique for lowering your arousal level over a short period, for example during a climb.

Once this is mastered it is possible to control other body functions such as heart rate and body temperature and thus raise and lower your arousal level at will. This technique is known as *autogenic training* and was first developed by a German, Dr Schulzt, and has been used to help patients with heart conditions, high blood pressure and other ills. This, like many relaxation techniques, is a very powerful tool and if you do suffer from any medical condition you should first consult your doctor before embarking on this type of training. To take autogenic training beyond the breathing stage we suggest you seek expert advice though you should be able to use it not only for short term relaxation such as in the middle of a pitch but also as an important element of planned relaxation sessions.

These sessions should take place after a training session preferably sitting up in a comfortable chair, since if you lie down you may tend to fall asleep and lose the quality of alertness. This will not matter if you are relaxing in order to bring balance back after a hard day or training session but if you are trying to relax in order to work on some mental training techniques then it is not suitable.

Progressive Relaxation

A second method which you may find preferable is known as progressive relaxation and was developed by an American, Dr Jacobsen. This technique involves alternately tensing and relaxing each muscle group in turn – starting with your feet and working progressively upwards – so that you can gain an awareness of each muscle group in a state of relaxation. As your awareness grows, you will increasingly be able to release all of the tension from your body and even, as recent research is indicating, different muscle groups at will whilst retaining tension in others. The implications of this for climbers are obvious.

A variation on the above is to lie on the floor (it can be done in a chair but it is usually easier to start by lying down) and to start by feeling all the areas that are in contact with the floor. Try to increase these areas, particularly the neck and back. Now again, starting with the feet, feel how the floor supports them, explore this feeling and you will find them feeling heavier and heavier. Now work up the legs to your thighs, then onwards when these feel heavy. Leave no part of your body untouched including the facial muscles, your tongue, your forehead, your eyes and your scalp. Now pause for a while and consider your thoughts and feelings then return to your feet and repeat the process again just to release the last traces of tension. Be aware that you can move at any time but choose not to because of the pleasure the relaxation is bringing to you. When you are ready stretch out and slowly get up. When you have mastered the technique of heaviness try, once the limbs are feeling heavy, to bring a sense of warmth to them.

There are of course many other methods such as the chanting of a mantra, yoga, or the technique of visualisation which we will deal with later. Closely linked with the skill of relaxation is the ability to concentrate and this too can be developed through training.

CONCENTRATION

You are on a climb which is at the limit of your ability but you are going well, the holds keep coming and you feel good. Suddenly you become aware that your last protection is twenty feet below you. It seems too far away now, as the tension invades your mind and you begin to feel the strain in your arms; you are getting pumped; your mind starts to race. 'Where are the next holds?' 'Where can I get some protection in?' A calm, balanced ascent has now turned into a fight for survival and all because something broke your concentration. The ability to concentrate is paramount to all sports and to many of life's situations in general. Concentration is the relaxed state of being alert so that you can maintain an awareness of all the changing information relevant to the climb at the expense of everything else. Training it can allow you to distinguish patterns of behaviour and thought that interfere, and may eventually let you change these.

In looking at how to improve concentration, we can use the climbing situation just described as an example. There are a number of ways to approach the problem. Try choosing a number of task-orientated thought patterns to use if a situation threatens your concentration. Focus on your breathing or focus on the next five feet of rock, looking at it intently, noticing its colours and shapes. This should be short and followed by the desire to climb on again (use visualisation to help train this response).

Alternatively, concentrate by deliberately paying attention to the distance from your runner and the emotion that it evokes, and agree with yourself that you will deal with it appropriately. You can play what could be described as the options game: What options are open to you? Can you place a runner without your strength running out? If the answer to this is yes, then do so, if not

you will just have to continue! Obviously this is very easy to say but a useful technique that can be used to help you to play this game is one known as the black box technique.

During a relaxation session after experiencing the above problem, picture the situation and then picture yourself at home at a desk or table. Write on a piece of paper the emotions and feelings you experienced, the ones that got in the way of the simple logic necessary to convince you to continue, fold the paper up and place it in a small black box which lives on the shelf next to the desk. Now return to your desk and think again about the climb and notice how much easier it is to cope with the situation. Finally you must return to the box, open it and read the things you wrote. They may in time no longer seem significant, which is fine, but it is important to give attention to these emotions because that is what you have promised a part of you that you will do. You should now be able to use this technique *in situ* (albeit in a shorter form so that it takes only a few seconds to have the desired effect), but again at the end of the pitch open the box and read the things you wrote. With practice many athletes have found this to be a very useful tool.

Concentration needs exercising so here are a few methods you could try. Take a picture of a climb or an object such as a karabiner, and when you are relaxed spend five minutes without moving, noticing as many qualities about the picture or object as possible. A similar exercise is to write down the name of an object connected with climbing. Draw a line out from this word like the spoke of a wheel and write down the first word that you associate with the original one. Return to the centre and repeat the exercise until you have a complete wheel.

There are any number of exercises that you could create to help with your ability to concentrate – perhaps the most important point is that you can improve it in just the same way that you can increase your strength or endurance. Like physical exercise it can be hard work and therefore needs the same dedication to achieve results. This same philosophy applies to the next area we will look at, visualisation.

VISUALISATION

The technique of visualisation, also known as mental imaging, is a very powerful tool in the field of mental training and has been used to great effect by many sportsmen and women in a wide variety of sporting situations. It most certainly has many applications for the climber.

We are all able to think visually but it is a considerable step from thinking with images to the technique of visualisation – like any skill it will take a period of dedicated practice before the benefits can be felt. If you do work at it, however, we feel sure you will find it beneficial.

Although we talk of visualisation it is important to realise that the images, the mental pictures that you create, should also include the other senses: your sense of touch, your hearing, your taste, and even your sense of smell. But why does picturing yourself doing a particular climb or sequence of moves help? To start with, the process of visualising an action actually sends a series of commands to the muscles involved and this will lead to a greater degree of control because not only are the muscles being activated but the nerve pathways are being used and the skill is being practised. Secondly, visualisation uses a language that the body can understand. Verbally describing an action can be very confusing compared to seeing it or feeling it.

Visualisation can also be used to help you to solve problems. The black box technique is one such application; another is to use it as a technique for helping you to relax. Sit in a chair and imagine you are full of a colourful liquid (choose your favourite colour). At your command you can let this liquid drain slowly from the ends of your fingers and toes. Turn these taps on and watch the level of liquid drop, first past your eyes, then totally out of your head and gradually onwards down through the rest of your body. Finally as the very last drops trickle from the ends of your toes you feel incredibly relaxed and totally supported by the chair.

When you are visualising a climb or sequence of moves the effect will be much stronger if you are relaxed and free from outside tensions. At the same time, however, it is important that you remain alert and able to concentrate as this will deepen the effects. If you realise that you are unable to concentrate for the whole period then it is best to shorten the session, a few minutes at a time is often sufficient. Your goals must be realistic – you should be seeing yourself performing at the best of your ability but not beyond its present state. It is no good seeing yourself floating up the hardest routes in the land when you normally climb in the middle grades. Use the technique specifically: imagine a particular sequence of moves and notice everything about them – the shape and texture of the holds; the ways in which your muscles tense and relax during the movement; the temperature of the rock; the direction the wind is blowing; the voices of other climbers; the colour of the rock; the sounds of the seagulls calling or the waves crashing if it is on a sea cliff.

Try to evoke all of your senses as this will make the images more powerful. For a long time it has been recognised that people tend to favour one sense over another when they are trying to absorb information – for most of us it is either the sense of seeing, hearing or feeling. When you start visualising, try to recognise which is the most dominant sense in your images and use this, adding the others later.

Not only will you find yourself having a bias towards one sense or another but also you may see yourself as from the outside, whilst others will feel that they are acting from inside themselves. Again work with whatever is the most comfortable to start with, but gradually try to work from inside yourself as this tends to use the kinaesthetic sense, which is the best sense to use when working on physical skills. Working from the outside in (using your visual sense) is also useful though, especially when you are trying to work out what is going wrong. Strange though it might seem, it appears that by viewing yourself from a short distance away you are often able to see what you were doing wrong more clearly.

As we said earlier, it is important to make your visualisation as realistic as possible and this means that it should take place in the present tense and at the correct speed. The only time when you might visualise at a slow speed is when you are picturing a particularly difficult series of moves where it is important to get it just right. Once you have established the sequence then return to the correct speed. Slow visualisation could also be of great use to those of you using 'dyno' moves. Run the move through in slow motion, paying particular attention to the hold you are going to grab. As you approach the hold see it clearly and sense that you have sufficient time to examine it before placing your fingers on it; feel as though you are able to float there momentarily. Now speed the sequence up but still retain the sensation of floating at the height of your 'dyno'. This may help you to feel as though you have more time to grab the hold, but it will also focus your concentration on the hold you are aiming for and away from other distractions.

As you have read this you may have noticed that you will have to have had previous experiences of the route before being able to practise the technique of visualising it. This is the key to the visualisation process – it needs practising as a technique before you can use it successfully in new situations. It should also be fun so that it remains positive. It is possible to visualise in a negative way and this of course is not desirable.

So far we have used visualisation to help rehearse moves and as you become more practised at this you will be able to use it on a climb just before embarking on a sequence. There are, however, other ways in which you can use this tool. Perhaps you appear to be having a bad day – take a few moments to remember a good day in the past and visualise it in detail, putting yourself back in touch with the feeling of performing well.

Use it to help you to relax in an otherwise tense moment, for example, holding on tightly with your right arm. After picturing the situation in detail focus on your right arm, feel the tension, feel the tightness of the muscles. Now turn to your left arm. The chances are that it too feels tight, so now relax that starting at the fingers and working down to your shoulders. Slowly work through the rest of your body, tensing the parts that are keeping you on the climb but relaxing the others. You may be tense because you are a long way from your last piece of protection. Tackle the tension and try to feel it drain away, leaving you in the same position but in a more relaxed manner, the same way that you would feel if you had been able to actually place some protection.

If your mental imagery will not allow you to feel this, replace the figure in the picture with someone you think could do what you are asking of yourself and then replace that figure with yourself again. In this example it does not even have to be another climber – you could, for example, if you were trying the above-mentioned 'dynos', picture the chimps at the zoo swinging effortlessly from branch to branch never missing the next hold. Now feel as though you are that chimp and perform the task: it will feel easy. Again replace the figure of the chimp with an image of yourself. This may sound comical but for many reknowned and respected sportspeople it has had astonishing results, so throw away your scepticism and examine the 'last performance frontier' of the modern athlete.

The ideas expressed in this chapter are not new or revolutionary, neither are they conclusive, as knowledge of mental training is constantly being expanded. They are, however, tried and tested and used to great effect in many situations, and they will, we hope, give you a taste for the potential that lies in this area of training.

Appendices

I SAMPLE PROGRAMMES

Individual climbers, quite rightly, view their training requirements differently, and the biggest mistake is to copy what someone else does in training simply because they climb well. Some people climb at a high standard regularly and do no training; others need to train hard and continuously in order to maintain their standard; some people train specifically for just one route, go and do it and then train for the next one.

We have interviewed a number of active climbers from a variety of countries, some at the top of the sport, others just enthusiasts, not to draw any conclusions but just to illustrate some of the points we are trying to make in this book. We have been pleased to see that since these interviews many of the participants have restructured their training programmes in an effort to make them more efficient. Our intention is not to be critical – we thank all those concerned for their contributions and apologise for any inaccuracies that may have occurred through the sometimes tenuous routes of communication.

Jerry Moffat (British)

Jerry does not feel he is a natural climber and attributes his standard to a carefully structured fitness programme. After nerve and tendon damage to the elbows in 1984 (as a result of overtraining) he stopped until 1986. He works on a 4-day cycle as follows:

1. Climb hard then train afterwards with weights and on ladders for power.
2. Rest.
3. Climbing – lots of bouldering, with training afterwards.
4. Rest.

He works on the upper body every fourth day with 2 sets of 3 reps (which means he is building his strength). He alternates muscle groups, writes down his progress and sets goals. He is not naturally supple and does some stretching. Generally healthy, and with a good diet, he has read about yoga and Zen but does not consciously use mental training techniques.

Geraldine Taylor (British)

Geraldine trains 4 days a week and climbs on the other 3. She has been training for the last 4½ years and has noticed a vast improvement as a result. She stretches for an hour every day and when she works on weights she usually uses 3 sets of 15 reps or a pyramid system. She orders her exercises rigidly and used to keep records, though she now feels that she knows her routines well enough not to bother. She takes care to warm up and down and uses mental training to psych herself up.

Jimmy Jewell (British)

Jim has been climbing for 15 years and has always trained. At the age of 18 he was a 400-metre runner. He is very powerful in the upper body and uses his feet well. He climbs and trains almost every day and in the winter spends 90 minutes, 5 times a week in the weights room and runs 7 miles twice a week. He uses 15 to 18 reps for most exercises with weights, with 3 × 6 for lats. He also does 200 pull-ups and 500 sit-ups, alternating in groups of 20 and 50 reps! Deltoids with a light weight are his favourite exercises and he usually does 5 × 100. A recent quote that Jim 'may not be able to pull on the smallest holds, but can pull up on those he can use all day' is reflected in this routine. He does very little warm-up and stretching, but warms down with light exercises. He does not keep records. He works on the climbing wall for forearms, and has some tendon damage in three fingers. Neurotic about his diet (at 6 feet, he weighs 10 stone 4 lbs), he keeps his weight down with a no-fat diet, mainly of fruit, vegetables and Ryvita, with no alcohol or drugs.

Tragically, since the writing of this book Jimmy has died. However, the authors feel sure that he would have liked his contribution to remain.

Todd Burroughs (American)

Todd has been climbing for 8 years but has only been training seriously for the last year. He uses ladders to train on, a method which is only beginning to gain popularity in Britain. He runs 3 to 4 times a week and uses his body weight in most of his routines, taking a minute's rest between sets. Although he keeps no records he does update his routine regularly. He stretches for ½ – 1 hour every day, warms up before exertion but does not warm down, and does some mental preparation.

Steve Haston (British)

Steve takes his training very seriously and has a good understanding of the principles of weight training, though his dead hangs are questionably dangerous.

Monday: rest day; 1/2 hours on flexibility.
Tuesday: warm-up and stretch, then climbing, followed by weight training. Shoulder presses: 5 × 8 reps. Dips: 5 sets. Pull-ups: 1 set of maximum, then 8 sets of half-maximum, then a hang till drop. Bent over rowing: 3 sets. Stomach curls: 3 sets. Forearm curls: 3 sets. (The number of reps in all of these sets varies from 8 to 25.)

Wednesday: rest day, walking and stretching.
Thursday: as Tuesday but with a variety of exercises on the weights.
Friday: rest, walk, stretch.
Saturday: climb 1 hard route. 2 hours kung fu, for stretch and reflexes.
Sunday: climb something very hard. No weights. 2 hours kung fu.

He prefers top roping for forearm strength and does a variety of finger and arm exercises of 3 – 5 sets with 15 – 25 reps.

Jean-Marc Kuyper (Swiss)

Jean-Marc runs 8 miles five times a week, and works out on weights and by using his body weight. He warms up but does not warm down. He stretches every time he climbs for about 10 minutes and his mental training techniques consist of visualising a beer at the top of the route!

Johnny Dawes (British)

Johnny has a rather unique physique and approach – he is very short, with sprinter's legs, not very obvious upper body strength, eats lots of chip butties (fried potato sandwiches) and hardly ever trains. However, he is extremely agile, has enormous dynamic energy and a very high degree of spatial (kinaesthetic) awareness. He can analyse the requirements of a pitch, compute the moves that will best get him up it, then move with great speed. Because he is short, John has developed dynamic moves to a fine art and will leap for holds he cannot reach, fully confident that he will stay on when he arrives. Currently he is developing 'second generation dynos' which involve the total removal of both hands at the same time, and he is also working on 'third generation' moves, where he uses a hold, which in itself is not good enough to hold on to, en route to the final one. This unusual combination of faculties and courage gives a unique climbing style.

Soviet Climbing Champions

Valery Balezin, aged 34, and Nadia Vershinina, aged 28, are the Russian champions of speed climbing. In the Caucasus and other areas climbing is a local pastime and scouts from climbing schools spot potential youngsters who are then taken to the climbing school for training. The competitions are on previously unclimbed routes, bolted for the competion. The climbers are seeded with the least experienced going first. Over a 50 – 60 metre route, Valery could watch other climbers go before him and estimate his own time to within about 10 seconds in 6 minutes. In the winter they train 6 days a week, cross country skiing, climbing in temperatures of −25°C, weights, and gym work. Their routines also contain components of flexibility and mental preparation, which they consider to be one of the most important elements (mostly a form of visualisation). Five weeks prior to the competitive season their climbing becomes intensive and very specific. All this is structured for them by trainers who pick their training routes and structure their days. There is little leading or placing of gear as all routes are bolted. They were both in fine physical shape, light, strong, supple and very careful with their diet.

Ron Fawcett (British)

Ron has been climbing and training for 16 years. Aerobic fitness and power training occupy more time in the winter and during bad weather. In the summer, weight training is for specific moves. Weight training sessions last for 1½ hours and are structured depending on current fitness. He keeps some records and does review and update weights and reps, depending on progress. He does 8 – 10 mile runs when the weather is unsuitable for climbing. He takes rest days quite seriously, is careful with diet and health (he is 6 feet 3 inches tall, and weighs 12 stone 2 lbs), stretches every day for 30 minutes, and certainly looks 'climbing fit'.

Freda Lowe (British)

Freda has been climbing for 20 years and is now becoming one of Britain's better women climbers. She does not structure her training but keeps herself aerobically fit by hill-walking. She has been attending stretching/training classes twice a week for the last 5 years. She uses the weights occasionally but does do fingertip pull-ups daily.

Randy Hershel (American)

Randy has been climbing for 5 years and training for the last 2. He runs 2 or 3 days a week, warms up and stretches for half an hour each evening and before climbing. He uses weights and body weight for his endurance training but does not keep records. He takes great care, as do most of the others, over his diet.

Nicky Wright (British)

Nicky has only been climbing seriously for the last 3 years but has made rapid progress. She trains mainly aerobically with a heavy emphasis on flexibility training which allows her to use her limited strength very efficiently. She attends stretching classes (which include some aerobic exercises) 3 times a week. Interspersed between these are occasional sessions with weights and she cycles on a regular basis. She does not keep records or set goals in her training.

These samples do show the variety of approaches to fitness training. There is no way everyone has to train, but for those who do want to, a lot of time and energy can be saved by structuring a programme which is tailor-made for you. You must be objective about your ability, realistic about your goals, and *want* to include training as part of your enjoyment of climbing. Then, with the knowledge gained within these pages, you should be able to construct a safe and efficient programme to suit your own special requirements.

II MUSCLES OF THE BODY

The following is a list of the major muscles in the body and the movements with which they are involved. The list is by no means exhaustive but nevertheless should prove helpful to you when you are trying to decide which muscles to work.

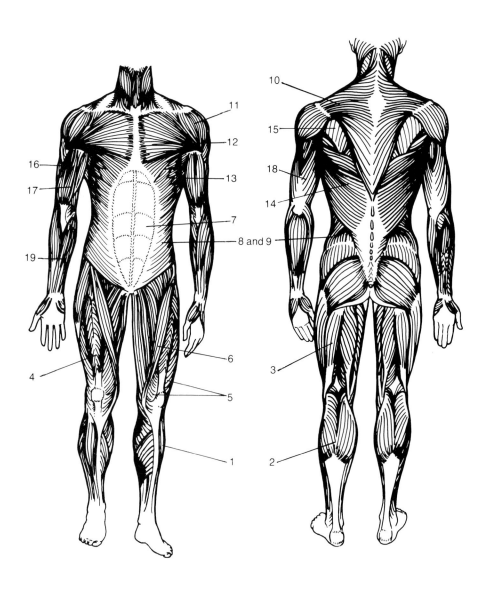

Fig 80 The muscles of the body (numbers refer to the table on page 91).

MUSCLE	ACTION	NOTES
Calf group		
1. Tibialis	Flexes the foot	
2. Gastrocnemius	Extends the foot but also helps to flex the knee	
Thigh group		
3. Biceps Femoris	Bends the leg and rotates the leg inwards	
4. Rectus Femoris	Straightens the leg and flexes the hip	
5. Vasti muscles	Straighten the leg	With the femoris, they form the quadriceps
6. Sartorius	Bends the leg, flexes the hip and turns the leg inwards and outwards	
Abdominals		
7. Rectus abdominus	Flexes thoracic and lumbar spine	
8. Obliques	Flex and rotate the trunk	
9. Transversus abdominus	Compresses the abdomen	Strong respiratory muscle
Shoulders		
10. Trapezius	Raises and lowers the shoulder girdle, moves the shoulder blades and head	
11. Deltoids	Raise arm to horizontal position	
12. Pectoralis major	Draws arm inwards, forwards and downwards, rotates the arm and helps to expand the chest	Important in pull-up manoeuvres
13. Serratus anterior	Acts in forward pushing and reaching	
Back		
14. Latissimus dorsi	Moves arm downwards and backwards	Important for climbing
15. Teres major, minor, Rhomboidus, and Infraspinatus	All assist with the raising and rotating of the arm and shoulder girdle	
Arms		
16. Brachialis	Bends the forearm to the upper arm	
17. Biceps	Bends forearm to the upper arm and turns the forearm	All of these muscles have obvious value to the climber
18. Triceps	Straightens the arm and draws it backwards	
Forearms		
19. Flexor and extensor carpi radialis, carpi ulnaris	Move the wrist	
Digitorum and pollicis muscles	Move the fingers and thumb	

III RECORD CARDS

Aerobic Training

On most activities it is possible to either increase the distance or reduce the time (italics) as you get fitter. Example figures have been included for your reference. However, you must work out your own when you start training.

SESSION	1	2	3	4	5	6	7
ACTIVITY							
Running							
Time (mins)	*30*			*30/27*			*30/25*
Distance (miles)	**3**			**3·2/3**			**3·5/3**
Fartlek (with stations)							
Stations (No. of reps)							
1 pull-ups							
2 curls							
3 press-ups	**10**			**10**			**15**[1]
etc.							
Time (mins)	*30*			*30/27*			*30/30*
Distance (miles)	**2·5**			**2·7/2·5**			**2·5/2·5**
Circuits							
Stations (No. of reps)							
1 press-ups							
2 curls	**10**/*10*			**15**/*10*[2]			**20**/*10*
3 shuttle runs							
etc.							
Time (mins)	*30*			**30**/*27*			**30**/*25*
No. of circuits	**3**			**3**			**3**

Notes:

[1] As you increase the number of reps so your times and distances will also adjust.

[2] Here we are either increasing the reps or reducing the time taken (italics). You could also include more stations or increase the number of circuits.

Strength Training

SESSION	1	2	3	4	5	6	7
EXERCISE							
Bench Press							
Max. wt or *RM(10reps)*	**70**/*50*				**75**/*55*		
Sets.	**3**				**3**		
Reps.	**10**				**15**[1]		
Kg (working wt.)	**50**/*25,40,50*[2]						

Notes:

[1] When you are able to increase the number of reps to 15 it is time to increase the weights.

[2] When using the *Repetition Maximums* system the first set should be at 50%, the second set at 75% and the third set at 100%. These too will increase when you are able to do 15 reps.

IV BIBLIOGRAPHY

Adams, G. *Designing a Fitness Training Programme*, The National Coaching Foundation, 1986.

Atha, J., and Wheatley, D. W. 'Joint mobility changes due to low-frequency vibration and stretching exercises', *British Journal of Sports Medicine*, 10, 1976.

Brooks, G. and Fahey, T. *Exercise Physiology*, Wiley 1984.

Cornelius and Hinson 'The relationship between isometric contractions of the hip extensors and the subsequent flexibility in males', *Journal of Sports Medicine and Physical Fitness*, 1980.

De Vries, H. A. 'Prevention of muscular distress after exercise', *Research Quarterly for Exercise in Sport*, May, 1961.

Gauron, E. F. *Mental Training for Peak Perforance*, Sports Science Associates, New York, 1984.

Gray's Anatomy, 35th Edition, Longman, 1973.

Hardy, L. 'Improving the active range of hip flexion', *Research Quarterly for Exercise in Sport*, 1985, Volume 56, No. 2.
'How can we help performers?', *Coaching Focus*, Autumn 1986, National Coaching Foundation.
'Active v. passive warm-up regime and flexibility', *Research Quarterly for Exercise in Sport*, 1986, Volume 57.

Harre, D. (ed.) *Principles of Sports Training*, Sportverlag, Berlin, 1982.

Harris, F. A. 'Facilitation Techniques', *Therapeutic Exercise*, 4th Edition, 1984.

Hay, J. *Biomechanics of Sports Techniques*, 3rd Edition, Englewood Cliffs, Prentice Hall Inc., 1985.

Hazeldine, Rex *Fitness for Sport*, The Crowood Press, 1985.

Holt, et al 'A comparative study of three stretching techniques', *Perceptual and Motor Skills*, No. 31, 1970.

Johns and Wright 'Relative importance of various tissues on joint stiffness', *Journal of Applied Physiology*, 1962.

Lamb, D.*Physiology of Exercise*, Collier Macmillan, 1984.

Liemohn, W. 'Factors relating to hamstring strains', *Journal of Sports Medicine and Physical Fitness*, 1978.

Matthews and Fox *The Physiological Basis of P. E. and Athletics*, 2nd Edition, W. B. Saunders and Co., 1976.

Matveyev, L. *Fundamentals of Sports Training*, Progress Publishers, Moscow, 1981.

National Coaching Foundation, *Physiology and Performance*, Coaching Handbook No. 3, 1986.

Orlick, T. *In Pursuit of Excellence*, Champaign III, Human Kinetics, 1980.

Pearl, B. and Moran, G. T. *Getting Stronger*, Shelter Publications Inc., 1986.

Railo, W. *Willing to Win*, Amas Export BV, Holland, 1986.

Roth, Darryl 'Climbers and Tendinitis: A Rehabilitation Approach', *Rock and Ice*, May – June, 1987.

Rowett, H. G. *Basic Anatomy and Physiology*, 2nd Edition, John Murray, 1973.

Rushall, B. S. *Psyching in Sport*, Pelham Books, 1979.

Straub, W. F. (ed.) *Sports Psychology: An Analysis of Athlete Behaviour*, 2nd Edition, Ithaca, New York, 1980.

Syer, J. and Connolly, C. *Sporting Body Sporting Mind*, Cambridge University Press, 1984.

Tancred, W. and Tancred, G. *Weight Training for Sport*, Hodder and Stoughton, 1984.

Tanigawa, M. C. 'Comparison of hold-reflex procedures and passive mobilisation on increasing muscle length', *Physical Therapy*, Volume 2, No. 7.

Weider, J. and Taylor, L. *Weight Training for Sports*, Sterling Publishing Co., 1985.

Williams, John G. P. and Sperryn, P. N. *Sports Medicine*, 2nd Edition, Edward Arnold, 1976.

Wirhed, R. *Athletic Ability and the Anatomy of Motion*, Wolfe, 1984.

Wright et al. 'Joint stiffness, its characterisation and significance', *Biomechanical Engineering* 4, 1969.

Index

OTHER CLIMBING BOOKS FROM CROWOOD

Hill Walking and Scrambling

Steve Ashton

This profusely illustrated book describes where to go, equipment, navigation, mountain weather, photography, basic ropework, and emergency techniques.

235 x 165mm   160 pages   ISBN 0 946284 58 X
143 photographs and diagrams plus 8 colour pages

Rock Climbing Techniques

Steve Ashton

With sound advice and expert instruction on the techniques of climbing, from movement on rock and rope methods to emergency procedures, this is an indispensable handbook for all rock climbers.

235 x 165mm   128 pages   ISBN 1 85223 228 5
139 photographs and diagrams plus 8 colour pages

Alpine Climbing

John Barry

A comprehensive handbook for the alpinist, offering extensive advice on equipment and the many skills required from basic rock climbing to advanced ice techniques.

235 x 165mm   208 pages   ISBN 1 85223 001 0
145 photographs, 88 diagrams plus 16 colour pages

Snow and Ice Climbing

John Barry

A fresh and informative look at this exhilarating game, covering equipment, skills, belaying and protection, starting out, and winter hazards.

235 x 165mm   144 pages   ISBN 1 946284 64 4
165 photographs and diagrams plus 16 colour pages

100 Classic Climbs

Essential guidebooks for the touring climber, illustrated with topo diagrams for each of the specially selected rock and ice climbs.

North Wales

Steve Ashton
ISBN 1 85223 020 7

Scotland (South & West)

Steve Ashton and Ken Crocket
ISBN 1 85223 025 8

Lake District

Stephen Reid and Steve Ashton
ISBN 1 85223 055 X

170 x 110mm   224 pages   plastic covers
route diagrams and photographs